The
Wisdom
of
Nurses

The Wisdom of Nurses

STORIES OF GRIT FROM THE FRONT LINES

Amie Archibald-Varley
and Sara Fung

Collins

The Wisdom of Nurses
Copyright © 2024 by Gritty Nurse Apparel Inc.
All rights reserved.

Published by Collins, an imprint of HarperCollins Publishers Ltd

First edition

This book draws on the experience of the authors and their interviews with other health professionals. Some names and other details have been changed.

HarperCollins books may be purchased for educational, business or sales promotional use through our Special Markets Department.

HarperCollins Publishers Ltd
Bay Adelaide Centre, East Tower
22 Adelaide Street West, 41st Floor
Toronto, Ontario, Canada
M5H 4E3

www.harpercollins.ca

Library and Archives Canada Cataloguing in Publication

Title: The wisdom of nurses : stories of grit from the front lines / Amie Archibald-Varley and Sara Fung.
Names: Archibald-Varley, Amie, author. | Fung, Sara, author.
Identifiers: Canadiana (print) 20230596355 | Canadiana (ebook) 20230596444 | ISBN 9781443468718 (softcover) | ISBN 9781443468725 (ebook)
Subjects: LCSH: Nursing—Canada. | LCSH: Nurses—Canada.
Classification: LCC RT61 .A73 2024 | DDC 610.73—dc23

Printed and bound in the United States of America
24 25 26 27 28 LBC 6 5 4 3 2

To my parents, Ian and Janny; my husband, Kevin; and my kids, James and Sadie, who inspire and encourage me on a daily basis.

—Sara

To my parents, especially my mom, who first showed me what grit truly means—and to my husband, Jordan, who unconditionally loves ALL of me, and our children (Logan, Tristan, and Emily), who make me a better person and mom every day.

—Amie

Contents

We (Really) Need Another Nursing Hero

Let's play a game. Name as many famous doctors as you can in a minute.

(And no, TV doctors don't count.)

How many did you come up with—five? ten? fifteen? Maybe some combination of names like Norman Bethune, Wilder Penfield, Sanjay Gupta, Anthony Fauci, Vivek Murthy, Atul Gawande, Theresa Tam, Elizabeth Blackwell, William Osler, Frederick Banting, Henry Morgentaler, Gabor Maté, Brian Goldman, Carolyn Bennett, Roberta Bondar . . .

Not a lot of women, but still—a good start!

Now let's do the same with nurses.

(. . .)

What's that? You need more than a minute? No problem! Take your time. We'll wait.

You only came up with one name, didn't you.

And that name was Florence Nightingale.

* * *

IT'S HARD TO think of any profession that is as completely dominated by a single figure as nursing is by Florence Nightingale. Many of you will know the broad strokes. Born in 1820 to a well-to-do English family in the city for which she was named, Florence Nightingale is considered by many the founder of modern nursing for her work caring for British soldiers in Turkey during the Crimean War (where she earned the nickname "The Lady with the Lamp" for carrying said lamp on her nighttime rounds), where her understanding of hygiene helped control and even reverse outbreaks of typhus, typhoid, and cholera.

For these and her other accomplishments, including the introduction of trained nurses into Britain's notorious workhouse system, and the use of statistical analysis techniques to reduce mortality rates in hospitals, Nightingale is treated with a reverence verging on adoration. The light coming off that lamp of hers might as well be a halo.

While other historical nursing figures have sparked and faded, the public continues to be reminded of Nightingale's legacy in myriad ways. Her life has been depicted in films, in books, in television, and on the stage. There's a Florence Nightingale award, a medal, a society, and a museum (in London, UK), and more statues, schools, and hospitals than you can shake a scalpel at. (There are four hospitals named for her in Istanbul alone.)

In fact, every continent on earth except Antarctica has something named after Florence Nightingale. And surely it's only a matter of time before Antarctica joins the club.

Nightingale was an avid gardener, so for the 200th anniversary of her birth, in 2020, the world-renowned Chelsea Flower Show deemed it fitting to create a garden in her honour (they named it "The Florence Nightingale Garden: A Celebration of Modern-Day Nursing"). The garden featured Nightingale's favourite bloom, the foxglove, as well as others found in her "extensive pressed-flower collection such as peonies and ferns, alongside other plants with strong healing properties like rheum (rhubarb), sanguisorba, and valerian, which were used in the nineteenth century and are still used in medicine today." Several flowers are also named after Nightingale, including a rose and a hibiscus described as "an unusual white flower with a large, deep red eye surrounded by lavender and pink rings."

Nightingale's imprint has extended beyond horticulture and medicine into the military realm. The cargo ship USS *Florence Nightingale* was used to land troops and cargo in North Africa during WWII, while the aircraft known as the C-9A Nightingale was used by the US Airforce for medical evacuation, passenger transportation, and special missions between the late 1960s and early 2000s.

Many nursing graduates in the US still recite some version of the so-called Florence Nightingale pledge, a modified version of the Hippocratic Oath, at pinning ceremonies. The original 1893 text reads:

> I solemnly pledge myself before God and in the presence of this assembly, to pass my life in purity and to practice my profession faithfully. I will abstain from whatever is deleterious and mischievous and will not take or knowingly administer any harmful drug. I will do all in my power to maintain and elevate the standard of my profession and will hold in confidence all personal matters committed to my keeping and all family affairs coming to my knowledge in the practice of my calling. With loyalty will I endeavor to aid the physician in his work and devote myself to the welfare of those committed to my care.

The pledge has since been modernized, and today most versions omit the cringeworthy parts about "purity" and aiding the physician in "his" work (insert eye roll).

WHEN IT COMES to Nightingale's efforts to inject science into nursing education, establish standards of care, and attend to the psychological needs of patients, her reputation largely still holds up.

In many other respects, not so much.

Although Nightingale died over a century ago, no one really seemed to question her legacy until 2020, when the New Zealand Nurses Organization (NZNO) announced that on International Nurses Day, which falls on May 12 and is—you guessed it—Nightingale's birthday, it would be celebrating Indigenous and home-grown nurses instead of Nightingale because of her "troubling role in colonization."

In New Zealand (and Australia), Nightingale had been a close advisor to colonial authorities, supporting the forced migration of Maori tribes so that European colonizers could settle their land and bring upon it "the inestimable blessings of Christian civilization."

In an outraged response posted shortly after the NZNO's announcement, Nightingale Society co-founder Lynn McDonald accused the NZNO of misconstruing Nightingale's language, and of failing to note that Nightingale had also called colonial rule "violent," "overbearing," "self-seeking," and "oppressive." In another post, titled "Florence Nightingale: A Leading Anti-Racist," McDonald said that the nurse "was the first person to make public the high rates of disease and death in residential and day schools in Canada."

But the NZNO's statement struck the louder chord, and a number of nursing websites and news outlets picked up on it. In November of that year, Dr. Natalie Stake-Doucet, an RN from Montreal, posted a much-read article, "The Racist Lady with the Lamp." Stake-Doucet referred to Nightingale's own writings—most of which are available online—to lay out some of the more problematic aspects of her legacy; in particular, her enthusiastic support of British colonialism, even when it involved the sacrifice of Indigenous people.

Stake-Doucet made it clear that her aim wasn't to erase Nightingale from the history books. Rather, she wanted nurses to better understand the figure they had been unquestionably worshipping for so long. "The historical figures we choose to venerate say a lot about who we are," she requoted from the NZNO's original statement.

HISTORY HAS TRADITIONALLY been written by victors and colonizers, so when we were first kicking around the idea of this book, we told our publisher we didn't want to knock Nightingale off the pedestal she's been on for so long—we nurses don't do violence—but at least to nudge her to the side of that pedestal. If we did that, we could make room for unsung or less-sung nursing heroes past and present. Maybe some nurses *without* the taint of white supremacy on them?

In a 2023 essay called "The Problematic Myth of Florence Nightingale," journalist Sarah DiGregorio explains what the effect of Nightingale's dominance of nursing history has been:

> The idea of Nightingale, the lady with the lamp, as the prototypical nurse—this mythic origin story—has served to further white supremacy in nursing and to strip nursing history of its truer, broader kaleidoscopic power. The real history of nursing is utterly radical in its vastness and in what it says about the care we owe each other. Maybe that radicalness is why that history has been so elided, even as nursing historians have sought to bring it forward.

If we could do that, then maybe we could help people see Nightingale for what she actually was: a deeply dedicated but also flawed and racist human being who was simply the most prominent in a long line of nursing achievers to come.

BUT THE TRUTH is that, initially at least, we struggled with our self-imposed assignment to find the revolutionary nurses, especially the *diverse* revolutionary nurses who were worthy of such adulation, the ones who could lead our profession as it continues to evolve in the twenty-first century.

Type "famous nurses" into a search engine and you might get three that aren't Nightingale or dead or American.

Search for "nurse influencers," on the other hand, and you'll get *lots* of names. But most are in the business of entertainment or self-promotion. They're not using the platforms they've built to advocate or create lasting change. They're more like caricatures of nurses.

So we turned, as we so often have, to social media. We asked our followers on Twitter (it was still Twitter then) to name nurses they admired from any era. Guess who almost everyone chose?

Those who didn't choose Flo usually went with a nurse they knew and liked but who had no real public profile. We were still at square one.

Near the end of *The Wizard of Oz*, Dorothy tells the new friends she made on the way to the Emerald City—the scarecrow, the tin man, and the cowardly lion—"If I ever go looking for my heart's desire again, I won't look any farther than my own backyard."

And it was in our own backyard—a.k.a. *The Gritty Nurse Podcast*—where we found the inspiring figures we were searching for, hiding in plain sight. People like Cathy Crowe (the OG!), Natalie Stake-Doucet, Dr. Leigh Chapman, Linda Silas, Ovie Onagbeboma, Carolyn Brost Strom, Renee Thompson, Nurse Blake, Tracy Zambori, Hadley Vlahos, Patrick McMurray, Ashley Bartholomew, Adrianne Behning, Jami Fregeau . . . (we're running out of breath!).

A few of those nurses, accordingly, are profiled in chapters of this book.

Mini-bios of other "Nurses with Grit" who we admire but haven't yet had a chance to speak to (or never will because they're dead) are sprinkled throughout these pages, names we think everyone should know.

As the profiles show, nursing has evolved radically since Florence Nightingale's day. No longer stuck exclusively at the bedside (although there are plenty of nurses who still love it there), today's nurses practise their science-based profession in a wide variety of ways and environments. For instance, community health nurse Debi Wade spends most of her time visiting clients in their homes, where she helps them find jobs or get their kids enrolled in school. As a pioneering street nurse, Cathy Crowe spent decades treating her dehoused clients in encampments, under bridges, and in shelters.

Then there are travel nurses like Swardiq "Q" Mayanja and Lindsay Pentland, who use hospitals' increased reliance on itinerant, short-term staff as an opportunity to see the world while making some decent cash.

Nursing has long been known as a "helping" profession, but Rachel Radyk showed us that help can come in different forms. In nursing school, Rachel started exploring and connecting with her Indigenous roots, and she has made serving that community the focus of her practice ever since. In doing this, she also attempts to shed light on some dark aspects of nursing history that many would prefer to leave in the cellar.

And of course there are also many, many nurses doing important work in clinics and hospitals. People like ICU and emerg nurse Nikki Skillen, whose rough exterior hides a heart of gold. Or David Metzger, a.k.a. Nurse Papa, who cares for children with cancer and wears his own golden heart right on his sleeve.

Then there are disruptors like Natalie Stake-Doucet, who channelled some of the lessons she learned from her hippie activist parents into getting what she needed to do her job properly during the pandemic.

INTERSPERSED WITH THESE stories are our own. Since we started our podcast in December 2019, we've become public figures and nursing advocates. We frequently get asked how we ended up in the profession, so we've shared our respective journeys in this book. Where did we come from, what first sparked our interest in nursing, what did we learn in nursing school? We describe experiences we've had while working in our specialties: labour and delivery (Amie) and postpartum (Sara). (Spoiler alert: some of the biggest challenges we face aren't patients but doctors and administrators.) You'll find out what *really* goes on during those infamous night shifts, how it feels when the tables are turned and we become the patients, and what it's like to do nursing on the fly.

Nursing is full of heartbreak and inspiration. It's also full of ghosts. Pretty well every nurse we've ever met has an uncanny story to tell. Many nurses will repeat these tales only to other nurses, but we decided to share some of these stories—plus a few of our own. (You're welcome!)

ANY OF THE nurses you meet in these pages could be a worthy successor to Florence Nightingale. But we believe that, collectively, we're an even greater force to be reckoned with.

Time for that old lamp of hers to shine its light forward.

Sara

*M*y *decision to go* into nursing was driven by my lifelong natural interest in health and biology. I remember, as an eight-year-old, pulling up a stool to my parents' closet so I could reach the anatomy books that were stashed on a high shelf there. They were boring, black-and-white textbooks with tiny print, not the gruesomely coloured ones with multi-layered transparencies you can pick up in bookstores, so I'm honestly not sure what the attraction was.

My mom had been a nurse, so to a degree I was also following in her footsteps. I say to a degree, because her prime motivation when she started nursing school was to be with my dad, who was studying engineering in Florida. They'd met by chance while she was down there visiting a friend who just happened to be my dad's roommate. Before that, Mom worked in a restaurant in Waterloo, Ontario, where she lived with her sister. My parents are both originally from Hong Kong, and like many immigrants who meet abroad, they quickly formed a bond, finding in each other a sense of comfort and belonging as they negotiated the new customs and traditions of their adopted home.

Other than a brief stint working the 3 to 11 p.m. shift as a bedside nurse, however, my mom never really practised. Language was a major barrier. My dad attended private school in Hong Kong and had a British tutor, so his English has always been pretty decent. But Mom grew up working class, and even though her English was never as bad as she thought it was, she still felt self-conscious about it.

The other problem was the job itself. Back in the '70s, bedside nursing was the only real option for nurses, career-wise, and my mom was put off by the profession's irregular hours, the lack of support for working parents—many of her colleagues struggled to find childcare during their shifts—and the patriarchal relationship that was then the norm between doctors and nurses. When she and my dad moved back to Canada, she decided to give up nursing and go back to work in the banking industry, which she'd done in Hong Kong and which interested her more anyway.

I was shy as a kid. So shy that in junior kindergarten they sent me for a hearing assessment because I wouldn't talk. I'm an introvert by nature. My default mode is to sit back and observe, but both my parents are the opposite. They're gregarious and have always been happy to do all the talking. Dad is someone who speaks with no filter, for good and bad. He's an interesting person who's been ahead of his time in a lot of ways, including his eating habits (he went low carb long before it became trendy).

My sense of shyness and the feeling that I was odd didn't benefit from the fact that my parents had what seemed like unusual jobs. In fact, I often had trouble explaining to friends what they actually *did*. Dad had an electronics-repair business that he ran out of our house. After reading everything she could about the stock market while working part-time at the bank, Mom became good at trading, which she did from home as well. Things are different today, but having a stay-at-home mom who did stock trading on the side did not seem normal in the '90s. (She still dabbles in trading. In 2021, she invested in GameStop during all the hype and managed to get out before it came crashing down. She's a really smart woman.)

It was in high school that I started coming out of my shell. Despite my shyness, I've always liked to try new things. This sometimes surprises people who associate curiosity with extroversion. But I like to try things quietly, on my own, with no announcements. I'll tell someone what I did after I do it.

I wasn't part of any clear-cut group or clique in school. I certainly wasn't an athlete. I joined the badminton team because there were no tryouts—they *had* to take me! And I wasn't a partyer, or maybe it's more accurate to say I never found out if I was a partyer because I never got invited to parties. No one ever offered me a cigarette either, I think because they assumed I wouldn't want one (I did).

I eventually found a happy place doing the morning announcements. Standing in the school office reading those daily scripts allowed me to be involved without feeling like all eyes were on me. I think this is part of why I like podcasting, too—it's funny how things can come full circle.

My parents were what many would consider typically Asian in their approach to child-rearing. They expected that I would get good grades, attend university, then find a respectable, predictable, well-paid job. You could say that going into a career where I helped others was in my blood. My paternal grandmother and aunt had both been social workers in Hong Kong at a time when it was rare for women to go to university, and they were proud of the years of service they provided to families of diverse backgrounds.

Still, what subject I should study post–high school felt, for a long time, like an open question. I liked English and biology (my biology teacher had been a nurse earlier in her career), but every other subject left me feeling indifferent. In the end, choosing nursing seemed practical. It was a job I figured my parents would approve of and that would give me a stable income.

But when I told my mom, she was pretty discouraging at first. Her brief but largely negative experiences as a nurse had led her to see it as a burnout job that I would soon want to quit.

Up until that point, Mom had always expected me to do what she told me to do. And generally speaking, I played the good little Asian girl and did just that (I'm an only child, which amped up the pressure a bit). But I was also starting to find my voice and feel like my own person, and I think I surprised her when I pushed back. Things are different now, I said. There were way more career possibilities in nursing than the bedside work she'd been stuck doing.

Although she eventually came round when she saw my excitement, my mom turned out to be right: I did burn out, though not for the reasons either of us imagined.

IN 2003, I ENROLLED in the four-year nursing program at the University of Western Ontario (later renamed Western University) in London, Ontario. I lived on campus, and even though all the students I met treated me like I was one of them, I felt like a fish out of water. An imposter. When we went around and introduced ourselves, it seemed like everyone had been class valedictorian except me.

For the next three years, it often felt like I had to work twice as hard as my classmates. I wasn't one to skip tutorials, and cramming before a test was too nerve-wracking. As a result of my study habits, by fourth year I had fairly good grades. More importantly, I passed all my clinical rotations and had largely gotten over my imposter syndrome.

I arrived at my own specialty through a process of elimination based on the rotations we did over three years. I quickly realized, for example, that mental health took a certain kind of person and that that person was not me. It seemed like a rotating door: people came to inpatient for treatment, got discharged, failed to take their meds, then ended up back in hospital for the same issue. It made me feel like I wasn't making a difference.

I tried hematology-oncology, but the placement left me feeling sad. So many patients didn't make it. Long-term care didn't suit me either. I wanted something more acute, though not as acute as emergency, which appeals to a particular kind of adrenaline addict that again, I knew I was not. (Emergency has other weirdnesses. Emergency room nurses often say, for instance, that they get patients who are more violent when there's a full moon.)

YOUR FINAL PLACEMENT in nursing school is called consolidation and involves working full-time for two to three months. Out of sheer luck mine happened to be in labour and delivery. I don't know how I got it. Every nursing student I knew wanted labour and delivery, but it's a lottery system. At Western, you listed your top three choices, but there was no guarantee you'd get any of them.

I was also aware that once you're in a specialty area, you usually stay there. When I started my consolidation in labour and delivery, I thought it was something I could really enjoy.

I had always imagined birth as messy, stressful, and medical (which it can be), but the first birth I attended was nothing like that. Everything was textbook. The mother was young, with no health problems, and was calm and in control throughout. The birth itself wasn't too quick or too slow. There was no sense of panic. The baby's heart rate followed a perfect, even pattern the whole time. There was barely any blood. The only surprising thing that happened was that the mother's water, which hadn't yet broken, came gushing out sideways when she was pushing, so I had to jump away to avoid it. (It helped me understand the importance of wearing waterproof shoes during births!)

The birth didn't just feel perfect, it was objectively so. Shortly after they're born, babies are assessed twice, at one minute and at five minutes, for their colour, heart rate, muscle tone, reflexes, and respiration. The resulting Apgar scores indicate how well they tolerated the birthing process, and how well they are doing outside the mother's womb, respectively. The physician at this birth assigned the baby an Apgar score of 10 on both tests and told me this never happened. I figured he was exaggerating but soon learned it was true: in all my years of nursing I have never seen two perfect scores again.

I was surprised by the flood of happiness I felt for this patient, a person who, before she came in, was a complete stranger to me. The whole thing was so beautiful I almost cried.

My preceptor was always trying to find interesting opportunities for me. One was attending a breech birth, where, instead of coming out headfirst, the baby exits the mother feet- or bum-first. I remember seeing the purplish presentation of the baby's bum, then the doctor reaching in and turning the baby around with all his might. There are very few doctors or midwives who have the skill to deliver breech nowadays, so it felt like a miracle to see this in action.

I was also present at a lot of unexpected, high-risk events: stillbirths, labours of mothers who were dealing with addiction, or who were precariously housed or homeless. It could be really intense, in good and bad ways. Sometimes at the same time. Once, during my consolidation in final year, I heard a patient thanking the obstetrician profusely for the way her birth had gone. It turned out that she'd been in a terrible car accident during her first pregnancy and had lost the baby. The impact had also ruptured her uterus. The doctor—the same one she was now thanking—had repaired it, allowing this birth to happen. The mother was ecstatic, despite what must have been quite a traumatic experience.

I learned how quickly and radically things can turn. A labour that seems to be going perfectly fine can change into an umbilical cord prolapse, a uterine hemorrhage, or an abnormal heartbeat requiring an emergency C-section. Labour and delivery is like an emergency in that it's predictably unpredictable (there's a lot of coordination between the two departments). It's not like other units, where the patient sleeps at night, giving you a chance to catch up on your work, or organize your supplies. In fact, labour and delivery is often busier at night than it is during the day. Unless a woman is induced, or comes in for a scheduled C-section, she doesn't control when she goes into labour.

One of my first jobs after graduating was in the postpartum unit at Mount Sinai, an academic teaching hospital in Toronto. I'd managed to nab a condo right across the street from the hospital, so getting to work couldn't have been more convenient.

My work in postpartum involved, among many other things, helping moms with baby care, breastfeeding, and getting their pain under control so they could go home. Interesting situations were always arising. For example, I once had a patient who was HIV-positive, which confused me, since her pregnancy appeared to have been naturally conceived and her husband was HIV-negative. She eventually admitted to me that she'd contracted the virus while having an affair. When she learned of her HIV status, she told her husband, and they began using protection, but somewhere in the window between contracting HIV and telling him about it, she got pregnant. I always wondered who the biological father of the baby was, but I guess it didn't matter. They were a happy family, all things considered. This and many other situations I would face taught me about the importance of staying impartial and focused only on the care required.

Being at an academic teaching hospital meant I got to see rare conditions and deal with patients from all walks of life, which was exciting and stimulating. There were always research studies going on and new techniques being tried—like giving infants small oral doses of sugar water to reduce the pain when they received heel pricks for blood collection. If I was assigned a patient with a condition I'd never heard of, I'd dive right in and research it as soon as I had the chance. I'd also try to talk to the patient about their diagnosis and how they managed the condition.

I later moved from postpartum to the neonatal intensive care unit (basically ICU for premature babies). In NICU, as it's known, there are different levels of acuity, Level 4 being the highest. I was in Level 3. People assume that because nurses "see it all," we become immune to the pain of others, but nothing could be further from the truth. We're nurses, but we're also human, and we can't help relating to what we see around us.

Honestly, I didn't anticipate the level of responsibility I would have in NICU. Once, when I was 26 weeks pregnant, I found myself looking after a baby who was the same age as my unborn child. The baby was on respiratory support and other life-saving equipment. It was a night shift, when there's not a lot of backup, and the baby's oxygen levels kept dipping down. It was stressful, and I found myself getting emotional. I kept thinking about how precious life is, how at any moment things can change. Nursing can send you on a rollercoaster ride. When the babies in my care were strong enough to go home, I felt great. But there were a lot that didn't make it. The reason could be as simple as an infection that made its way to the bloodstream—which is way more common than you'd think. It was something I never got used to. I met mothers who had had multiple losses, or who'd gone through the difficult process of getting pregnant with IVF, only to have their baby end up in the neonatal ward. We once had a baby die on Christmas day, and I remember the mother came in and just collapsed. She thought her child had died because of something she had done—she blamed herself, in other words. The woman was new to Canada, and her life was clearly already difficult. The next day she had to take a bus home all by herself, which broke my heart.

It was in the NICU that I really came to understand what an impact we nurses can have on patients. Even a fleeting daily interaction, whether it's helping new parents learn to bathe, diaper, or feed their baby, or offering a shoulder to cry on or a hand to hold can mean a lot. On stressful days when we were short-staffed, it made me happy to know that my work was appreciated. I might become part of someone's life story after, let's say, delivering the news to a mom who had had a pregnancy-loss scare that her baby made it. Parents would sometimes show up on the ward asking to see the nurses who delivered their babies twenty-five years ago.

Once, when I was taking care of a patient in a semi-private room in postpartum, a voice suddenly called out from the other side of the curtain: "Sara?" It turned out to be a woman who'd been in one of the prenatal classes I taught. She was at the hospital having her second baby, and she seemed incredibly happy to see me. She said she'd been wanting to thank me for all the useful advice I gave her before the birth of her first child. She had used no epidural and was planning the same for her second. It's at times like these when I realize the impact we can have on patients' lives. It's an impact that's difficult to gauge because we often don't see patients after they leave our care, especially when it's in the hospital.

Of course, the reverse is also true: Nurses have stories we tell over and over again about patients who touched us in a way that we will never forget. Ones that make us feel like we truly make a difference.

But as meaningful as the work at Sinai often was, after eight years it started to feel like something was missing. I've always liked challenging myself. So I finished my master's and joined every committee I possibly could. I did research and teaching stints outside the hospital and even worked at a women's health clinic. Wanting to bring about change, to use my research skills in new projects, I applied for jobs I was qualified for, but I never got hired. It seemed like there were no more opportunities for me to move up, at least not where I was.

I eventually found a position as a clinical nurse specialist (CNS) at a hospital outside the city. CNS is what's called an advanced practice or leadership position, since it requires a master's degree. My time would be split between working by the bedside and making quality improvements to the unit as a whole. Specifically, I'd be responsible for creating new emergency codes and care plans for high-risk patients with complex medical conditions and social challenges, such as domestic partner violence or substance abuse. The job would allow me to have a positive impact not just on individual patients, but on the entire Maternal Child Program at two hospital sites. This appealed to me deeply.

However, I'd spent so much time wanting to get to this level that I initially felt the way I had back in my first year at nursing school: like an imposter. I was in awe, intimidated by everyone around me.

In nursing, experience is emphasized over other accomplishments, such as education. Ask any nurse about their career and the first thing they'll talk about is their years of experience and the jobs they've held. It's very different from fields like the tech industry, where being young and cutting-edge is seen as an asset. Nurses typically start taking on a leadership role somewhere in their forties, or after at least twenty years' experience, whichever comes first. I was only thirty—it was unusual that I had done my master's degree directly after my undergrad—and as a result my colleagues treated me as if I didn't have the "street cred" to lead. (I've also always looked younger than I am, which I realize is a good problem to have, most of the time!) When I talked about improvements I wanted to make on the unit, some colleagues would visibly roll their eyes. Others questioned me in a hostile manner, asking if I had the credentials to do what I was doing. It felt like outright bullying. This was a relatively small non-teaching hospital, and I got the sense that the nurses felt threatened, that they believed I thought I was better than them because I came from one of the "fancy" urban hospitals that got all the funding. The worst thing was that I hadn't been introduced to staff when I came to the unit, so I had no one to talk to about what I was experiencing, no one to back me up.

The population my team would be servicing was high-needs, both financially and health-wise, and my responsibilities would include, among other things, educating nurses, implementing practice guidelines, and writing policies. Physically I would be on the ward, but in an office. If there was a Code Pink—when a baby isn't breathing, for example— my role would be to support the staff by doing crowd control, documenting the incident, explaining to family members in real time what was happening in layman's terms, and debriefing staff afterwards.

I'm not a negative person, so it was hard for me to acknowledge that almost from the start, the job wasn't what I expected. The bureaucracy and the politics were crazy. Initially, it seemed like there would be opportunities to improve things, especially with projects I'd be starting from scratch. So it confused me that I was not given the information I needed to transition into the job properly.

For example, I was supposed to conduct reviews of cases in which the outcome for the mother or the baby hadn't been good. But I couldn't get access to any of the relevant files. Instead, I was told I was not on the unit often enough, even though they knew I could only be there two days a week since I worked at the other location the other three. Sometimes a staff member would accept my request for a meeting, but then either not show up or take calls during it. Due to lack of space, I didn't have a dedicated office area, so at one point the hospital's lactation consultants kindly offered me a desk in their room. I later learned that people were being told that I never worked, I just "hung out" with other staff in the office all day. Someone even made negative comments about my physical appearance that made me very uncomfortable.

It felt like I'd been given all the responsibility for making change, but none of the resources. I was being undermined at every turn. My "dream job" soon started to feel unproductive and frustrating.

A case in point was policy writing, which was supposed to be a major part of my role. Individual hospitals have a huge number of policies, which have to be updated every two years. It's like painting the Golden Gate Bridge: as soon as you're finished, it's time to go back and start at the beginning again. Some of the work is straightforward and involves following a decision tree or an algorithm like a series of predetermined steps. Other policies concern specific procedures. In maternal care, for example, there are policies about the time it takes to do a C-section when baby and mother are in distress. If a baby's heart rate is decreasing, doctors must adhere to a standard based on timelines associated with best outcomes. There are policies for when labour should be induced, and what steps to take during a Code Pink. The policies themselves are usually based on data and findings from outside pediatric or obstetrical organizations. As nurse leaders we needed to keep abreast of these ever-changing guidelines and incorporate them into our hospital's own policies. Updating policies also requires getting approval from all the stakeholders involved, from doctors to nurses to managers to midwives—even security—which involves committees and many time-consuming meetings (so many meetings!).

Once a policy is created, the next step is to make sure everyone is aware of it. This might sound straightforward, but it can quickly become unmanageable. Doctors, for instance, often have ways of doing things that they expect will be reflected in the policy. I soon discovered that if this wasn't the case it could result in a power struggle. Physicians aren't actually employees of the hospitals where they work, but they do have privileges. And because they don't report to a manager or a direc-tor but to a department head who is a fellow physician, doctors don't even have to abide by the policies they're presented with. Sometimes, we'd go to a hospital with our finished policy and the management would just go ahead and change it right in front of us. In the end, my experience working in policymaking left me feeling disempowered and highlighted how inefficient healthcare can be.

A QUICK WORD on doctors. We've moved away from the era when you had to give a doctor your chair when he (back then it was almost always a "he") came into the room. But how your day goes as a nurse still depends very much on who's on call—doctors are in charge for up to 24 hours at a time—and specifically, what their mood is.

In some hospitals the culture is more collaborative; in others it's more authoritative. Academic teaching hospitals are, by nature, more used to dealing with research and innovation, whereas staff in community hospitals are less accustomed to people cycling in and out. In my experience, it can be harder to work with physicians in community hospitals, where there tends to be a bigger power differential in relationships, and where change is sometimes met with resistance. We nurses spend the majority of our time at the bedside, connecting with our patients, so if we voice concerns and nothing changes, it can make us feel powerless. On the other hand, when a doctor treats us as what we are—the eyes and ears of a hospital—it incentivizes us to say what's on our minds so that we feel like we make a difference.

Another thing that frustrated me about my leadership job (which, I might add, had previously been performed by two people) was that it was spread between two hospitals, both of which complained they didn't see me enough. It was only recently, when a third hospital tried to get me to work there as well, that I finally put my foot down.

Which isn't to say the experience was all bad. On the positive side, I was working with a small group of leadership nurses who really supported one another, one of those nurses being Amie. And there are things I accomplished in that position that I'm really proud of. One of my biggest assignments was getting the hospitals' breastfeeding rates up—they'd hired me, in part, because as a trained lactation consultant I had expertise in breastfeeding. I organized a 20-hour non-mandatory course to educate nurses about breastfeeding. It encompassed issues like alternative feeding methods, how to intervene in difficult medical situations, and how to be non-judgmental of mothers from diverse backgrounds. The feedback was really encouraging. Most of the nurses who took the course came away feeling empowered by it. It eventually became so popular that we couldn't accommodate everyone who wanted to enroll.

The city where I was working was very diverse: 73 percent of the population were visible minorities, primarily of South Asian (mostly

East Indian), Black, and Filipino descent. So I had posters made with information about breastfeeding in Punjabi, Urdu, and Gujarati. We put these up in patient rooms, toilet stalls—anywhere we thought mothers and mothers-in-law would see them. (One thing I learned is that in many South Asian families the mother-in-law has a *lot* of say in baby care, so if you can get to her, often you can make a difference.) The idea was to remove as many barriers to breastfeeding as possible for every patient who came through the hospital, and to understand why breastfeeding might not be their first choice.

I stayed in that position for almost two years, until I went on maternity leave for my second child. Knowing that I wanted a change when my mat leave was over, Amie recruited me (at different points in our careers we've been on each other's hiring panels, which is cool) to work alongside her in a brand-new hospital in an affluent city farther west. We had shared an office before and had gotten along really well. But we had also been a bit like ships in the day, more acquaintances than colleagues. In this new placement, we would be working for a year in the same office, essentially in the same role but covering different units. The hospital was state-of-the-art, and I was in a condition of near-euphoria. Unlike in my previous position, here we had resources, nurse colleagues who were interested in making a difference, and doctors who supported us. Was this, finally, my dream job?

Far from it, unfortunately. And my—or in this case, our—biggest challenge turned out not to be the work. It was an issue that was more interpersonal.

Right from the outset, we faced unrealistic expectations of what we could accomplish in the time we had been given. For example, shortly after I started, I was asked to uprate and create a new decision algorithm to manage infants that had hypoglycemia (low blood sugar) after birth. I was to accomplish this in 90 days, even though it would require approval from three hospital sites and would involve upwards of a hundred stakeholders. I knew from experience that six to nine months was a more realistic timeframe.

The longer it took, the more frustrated they got with me. But they kept laying on the work, and the stress kept building. At some point I started pushing back, telling them that what they were asking for was unreasonable, but they kept wanting more and more. Here's an example: To educate nurses on changes that were coming, I was asked to evaluate them during fake emergency situations (called mock codes), which we would organize and run. But the nurses weren't given dedicated time for this. Rather, they were expected to somehow undertake these role-playing scenarios *while* they were working.

Another time, when we were showing nurses how to ration infant eye ointment due to a national shortage, they wanted the new policy written in days, essentially an impossible task, unless you're willing to cut corners on the normal hospital process, which they weren't. It usually takes months to properly draft new policies and get them approved.

When my instructions were unclear, which was often, and I asked for clarification about what I should be doing, the usual response was to throw the question back at me: "What do *you* think you should be doing, Sara?" Not helpful.

Then came the gaslighting. I'd tell them what I was working on, and I'd be told, "This isn't what we discussed." Wait, what? Luckily, I had taken notes during that discussion, or I would've thought I was going crazy. And when things didn't go right, they'd immediately look for a scapegoat. I didn't feel comfortable responding that I'd simply been carrying out the project that I was assigned, but that was the truth. It was as if we were being set up to fail. And the pressure was relentless.

I had landed in another situation where I simply couldn't do the job I'd been hired to do, despite the fact that I was both capable and eager.

But this time I had Amie to bounce off of. She too was attempting to balance a ton of projects with limited resources.

In leadership, however, you can't get away, and I often felt trapped and bullied. This is the conundrum I was in.

Amie and I both felt lost, like we didn't have a voice, let alone a platform to share experiences. We didn't know it at the time, but these days would cement the experiences that led to the podcast.

I WENT TO see my family doctor. Once I was in his office, I broke down. He told me I needed to take stress leave. But in a kind of Catch-22, I couldn't get time off without a psychiatric diagnosis, which would take six to eight months. I did see a therapist; although she couldn't give me a diagnosis, she was able to treat me.

I ended up taking unpaid leave for almost a month. During this time, Occupational Health, the department that makes decisions about work leaves, kept asking me to fill out more forms. At one point I asked outright if my job was secure. (If I had been a bedside nurse, I would have had a union supporting me, but most nurse leader positions are non-unionized.) In the eyes of Occupational Health, I was simply refusing to come to work, despite the fact that in my entire working life I'd never taken any time off other than maternity leave. In the end, instead of getting stress leave, I got a crash course in the problems plaguing the mental health system.

Under pressure, I returned to work. But nothing changed. Management didn't relieve me of any of my workload, which was a major source of the stress. All the time I spent filling out forms during my "leave" left me feeling like I'd had no respite at all. Maybe if I'd stayed at the job longer something would have come of my case. But after eleven months, the hospital no longer felt like the right place for me. So in October 2019 I did the only thing I felt there was left to do and resigned. Amie had done the same a month earlier.

BEFORE WE RESIGNED, Amie and I had been in a kind of denial. We didn't want to believe what was happening to us. We had, after all, come to this hospital from jobs where we were both unhappy. It was disillusioning, frustrating. We'd been naïve enough to believe that if we took our concerns up the chain of command something would happen. It didn't. Ultimately, I think management was grateful that we moved on to other jobs and didn't escalate our concerns.

Two negative experiences in a row convinced me that I needed to work outside of a hospital setting, and a month later I landed a job at a homecare agency doing community care in downtown Toronto. Like the other nursing leadership positions I had held, this one would involve education, policy writing, and special projects. Working out of the organization's corporate office, I would be in charge of education and quality improvement projects for nurses and personal support workers (PSWs). I was nervous.

I don't know if it was because there were no physicians, because we had a more balanced gender- and racially diverse team, or because I was finally out of the hospital system, but right from the get-go I loved the work culture at my new placement. I'd become accustomed to bad work practices, like acquiring needed information through gossip. Here, refreshingly, there appeared to be no hidden agendas, no one trying to undermine me: we simply got things done. When a problem arose, we dealt with it instead of finding someone to blame. I was working with a team of about ten, which was smaller than what I was used to, and possibly that streamlining resulted in fewer power struggles.

There were other differences. In hospitals, nursing leadership is typically dominated by women. Now, for the first time in my nursing career, my boss was a man, and I found his approach new and innovative, including his embrace of technology to streamline training and other processes. The office was mostly paperless, and we worked from home one day a week well before the pandemic.

In my previous two positions, I spent so much time on bureaucracy and politics, figuring out who I should talk to, that there was no space to improve things. I was just trying to keep my head above water, to say the right thing to the right person. Now all those issues seemed to have magically vanished, and I even managed to find the personal healing time I felt I needed. It required a pay cut, but it was worth it.

I LEFT THAT job reluctantly, but on good terms, in 2022 to start a business doing career coaching for nurses. By then Amie and I were doing the podcast, which she had suggested shortly after we both quit our jobs in the fall of 2019. I didn't really listen to podcasts, but I'm always willing to try something new, so I thought, "Why not?" We got some advice from Amie's cousin, who had a podcast, and I found YouTube videos that explained the technical requirements, which at that point looked like it was going to be the hardest part.

One of our earliest episodes, a three-parter about nurses' experience of bullying, was therapeutic for both Amie and me. In other episodes we talked about the quirks of nursing, the funny little things we thought other nurses would understand, the crazy night-shift stories, the difficult patients. Mental health issues became a mainstay of the show, as well as advocacy, which we quickly came to feel passionate about.

Once in a while I'll google nursing news on my phone, and the algorithm feeds me an article I've written or a TV or radio spot I was on. But the truth is I still find live interviews a challenge. There are no do-overs; sometimes people go off-script and ask questions you weren't anticipating. I've learned to adapt to this in the moment, and Amie's cousin has shared useful tips on shifting the conversation back to a comfortable spot. I still don't listen to any other podcasts regularly—occasionally I'll listen to another nursing podcast—for the simple reason that I don't want to compare myself to anyone else!

One of the reasons Amie and I work so well together is that we're opposites personality-wise. Amie's an extrovert, a relationship-builder. When I came to work at her hospital, she introduced me to everyone. And she plays the same role on the podcast: she networks to get people on the show, while I handle logistics, scheduling, and finances (not that we thought about any of this when we started). When Amie is passionate about something, she's all in, and people respond to that. It's a quality that draws people to the podcast too.

I used to find my parents' work lives perplexing, but these days they're the ones who don't understand what *I* do. Advocacy isn't something I grew up with. My new career path isn't one they can relate to, but they're still trying to understand it. Asian culture, in particular Chinese culture, is very focused on practicality and minimizes the importance of creativity. Technology intimidates my parents, so they haven't listened to the podcast much. This used to upset me, but I've learned that you can't expect your friends and family to tune in, at least not to every episode. And of course, the upside is that I can talk about my parents on the podcast (which I do) without worrying about hurting their feelings. All this isn't to say my parents don't support us. When Amie and I were on the front page of the *Toronto Star* they bought lots of copies. They are particularly proud of my published articles, especially since *Chatelaine* was a mainstay in my house when I was growing up. Seeing me on the news also surprised them and filled them with pride. And they were clearly proud when our extended family began calling and emailing them, telling them what a great job I'd done, after they saw me on the news. My dad always has lots of opinions to share with me, but he's also a very private person. He seemed impressed that I was discussing my opinions in such a public way.

The podcast has led to another change in my relationship dynamic with my parents, a mostly positive one. In 2021 I moved from Toronto to Hamilton, where they lived, so we could be closer, and so they could see their grandchildren more easily.

My nursing career didn't go the way I expected, and yet I've never regretted the path I took. If things had gone differently, I wouldn't be the person I am now. (My only regret is that I didn't tell the people who caused me so much grief the real reason I left my job, which was that I was barely holding myself together emotionally. The environment was just too stifling.) Despite the ups and downs, nursing has given me confidence. I finally feel like a leader, even if it's not the kind of leader I imagined when I went off to do my master's. It's hard to reconcile Sara the public advocate with the little person I used to be. The kid who wouldn't talk does an awful lot of talking these days.

NURSE WITH GRIT

Mary Seacole (1805–1881)

Like Florence Nightingale, Mary Seacole worked as a nurse during the Crimean War, where she set up quarters for sick and convalescent officers that became known as the "British Hotel." For a time, she was almost as famous as Nightingale, being dubbed, in contrast to "The Lady with the Lamp," as "The Creole with the Tea Mug" for her habit of providing hot tea, cake, and lemonade to wounded soldiers awaiting transport to hospital.

Born in Kingston, Jamaica, Seacole's Scottish father was a lieutenant in the British army, and her mother a free Black "doctresse," who used a combination of modern hygiene and traditional Caribbean and African herbal medicines to treat members of the community. Seacole's autobiographical account of her extensive travels, *Wonderful Adventures of Mrs. Seacole in Many Lands*, is considered the first autobiography written by a Black British woman (Jamaica having been a British colony at the time). In contrast to Nightingale, Seacole died in poverty. By the time of her death in 1881 at age seventy-one, her name had been nearly forgotten. But she has experienced something of a revival in the years since, with buildings, statues, hospital wards, and prizes now named for her. In 2004, she was voted number one in an online poll of 100 Greatest Black Britons, created following the backlash to a previous list, 100 Greatest Britons, that included no Black Britons at all. (On that list, Florence Nightingale clocked in at number 52.)

Salman Rushdie wrote a line about Seacole in his 1988 novel, *The Satanic Verses*, that succinctly sums up her legacy: "See, here is Mary Seacole, who did as much in the Crimea as another magic-lamping lady, but, being dark, she could scarce be seen for the flame of Florence's candle."

Amie

A lot of the nurses I've met tell me that they knew what they wanted to be from the time they were little. Not me. My nursing journey has been far from a straight line. As a kid growing up in Brampton, Ontario, my first dream was to be a weather girl like the one I saw on *Global News* early in the morning before *Care Bears* and *Inspector Gadget*. I'm not totally sure why, although the performative aspect definitely appealed to me. I was also fascinated by sciences from an early age.

I was always gregarious, opinionated, out there. I liked my voice to be heard. I was insatiably curious too. My mom called me her little elephant, because wherever she went, I was always right there next to her, and because I was *loud*. Our home was conservative and religious, however, so when my curiosity pertained to sex and sexuality, it didn't go over all that well. In my West Indian parents' eyes, sex was for marriage and procreation only—or so they wanted me to believe.

When I was younger, I dutifully attended our Pentecostal church every Sunday. The church itself was small and homey, but later, as the congregation grew, it moved to a building more akin to an amphitheatre than a traditional church. The facility, which easily accommodated 500 people, was beautifully lit, with a central stage framed on either side by large screens that displayed hymn lyrics and eye-catching graphics. The music was upbeat (similar to that produced by Hillsong Church, before the latter became famous, then notorious). The atmosphere was outwardly friendly and warm, and yet from an early age I sensed something else. An underlying sense of judgment? I could tell some parishioners were insincere, going through the motions for show. When I was seventeen, I stopped attending services regularly. It was less difficult than I had thought it would be. If I just slept in, Mom, who was always in a rush to get out the door, simply let me be.

The baby of the family typically has it the easiest, but in my case, it was the opposite. My parents were a lot harder on me than on my brother, Lenworth Jr., or my sister, Shelleen. I've never been one to beat around the bush, so I'm going to say right out here that in my experience there's a lot of misogyny and sexism in Caribbean culture. Boys are expected to get into trouble, girls to be polite and demure. My father's unspoken expectations were that I, like all women and girls, should cook, clean, and serve men. But I wasn't demure or subservient. Far from it! And I pushed back. This led to a breakdown in my relationship with my father that was difficult for my mom. Loving but firm, she found my inquisitive nature overwhelming and refreshing at the same time. I got the sense that she felt torn between wanting to let me be "free" and acceding to my dad's demands.

I wasn't only curious about sex and reproduction. Physical objects intrigued me as well. I was one of those kids who loved to take things apart and see if I could put them back together again, a habit that, as you can imagine, wasn't too popular with my parents. When I was eight, I managed to get my hands on a delicate gold watch my grandma had bought for my mother on a trip to England. Mom had seen me with it earlier in the day and, knowing my disassembling habit, warned me more than once to leave it alone. I smiled and told her I just wanted to appreciate its beauty—which I did . . . by taking it apart. I grabbed a miniature screwdriver and hid behind our pink velour couch (it was the '80s, and dusty rose was all the rage in West Indian décor). I remember my sense of fascination as I examined the watch's various components, the tiny bolts and screws, the way they were all interconnected. Since my mom will be reading this book, I won't outline exactly how she handled the situation. Let's just say that I never did anything like that again.

The childhood habit of asking questions stayed with me and has mostly stood me in good stead. Mom spent a little time at university, but I'm the only one of my siblings to complete post-secondary school. In my first year as a nurse, I discovered that the single most important question you can ever ask is: How can we do things better?

I COME FROM a big, loving—albeit complicated—family. My mom is one of thirteen kids (although sadly, three died) and my maternal grandparents, Maxwell and Ivy Shepherd, were patriarch and matriarch. They were the first members of our family to come to Canada. My parents were both born on the beautiful island of Jamaica: Mom on the north side, in St. Mary's; Dad on the south side, in Clarendon. In typical immigrant style, they met in Canada, specifically Toronto, through Mom's younger twin brothers. Dad was working as an un-licensed mechanic (he later got his licence, thanks to much dedication and to my mom, who walked him through the exam), and Mom had a job at an insurance company. Before she met Dad, Mom lived for a few years in Montreal, where she worked as a model.

After they married, my parents bought the little townhouse in Rexdale, a community northwest of Toronto, where I spent the first two years of my life. In 1986, when gang-related crime was on the rise in the area, my alarmed parents packed up and moved us slightly west, to Kingswood Drive in central Brampton. I loved it there, partly for the convenience: our house was literally in front of my elementary school. The bell would ring, and I'd run right across the street to class. We had one of the biggest houses on the street, a corner lot with a gigantic maple tree and a huge side-yard and backyard. I have warm memories of that time: playing with friends, going to the local Becker's, and riding my bike along sunny pathways on endless summer days.

Kingswood, contrary to what that last anecdote might suggest, wasn't all rainbows and unicorns. As I said before, I was a very open and friendly child. Skin colour wasn't something I consciously thought about, especially within my family, which encompassed a variety of cultures: West Indian, East Asian, European, South Asian; we were a big, beautiful blend! So I was completely shocked when, at age seven, I approached a group of white boys to ask if they wanted to play and one of them answered, "We don't play with n***ers." I had only heard this word once before, in the movie *Rosewood* (my parents were watching it late at night, and I'd snuck downstairs to see what this whole "restricted movie" thing was all about). It didn't make sense. Why would someone hate me, or anyone else for that matter, because of the colour of our skin? My brother and sister, who were nearby and overheard what the kids had said, stormed over. I remember being amazed at how quickly their moods changed. They loomed over the boys, said something my parents would certainly not have approved of, and whisked me back home. I will never forget the look of deep hurt on my mom's face and the tears that rolled down her cheeks when we told her what happened.

Though this would not be the last time I experienced racist abuse and harm, I never got used to it. Every single incident was painful in its own way. When you're young you don't expect others, particularly adults, to behave like that. You assume an ugly encounter is just a one-off, or, if you're Canadian, that racism is more of an American problem.

It was only when I was older that I learned about systemic racism and how pervasive and insidious it is, including in my country, Canada. My parents never became comfortable talking about sex, but like many Black families we had the "race and racism" conversation early. In my case it was right after that incident with the white boys. My mom had never known racism personally until she came to Canada at eighteen. She got a job at a Toys R Us store, where the white woman who was training her called her a "Jungle Bunny." She had white co-workers who wouldn't look at her or address her when she was in the room. After meeting my mom's mother, Grandma Shepherd, one co-worker even asked Mom if she was "adopted." (My mother has dark skin, but Grandma Shepherd, who was West Indian with some Syrian ancestry, was "white passing.")

Grandma Shepherd had been a nurse in Toronto. I remember her talking about the racism she'd seen at work; how the white nurses would say horrible things to her about Black patients, not realizing she was Black. I don't know why those stories didn't change my mind about going into the profession. Maybe subconsciously they solidified my resolve. I've always been a fighter.

My maternal grandfather, Grandpa Shepherd, was a bombardier in Britain's Royal Air Force during World War II. I used to love hearing his stories about comradeship and his feats of bravery. He often went to the Canadian Legion to reminisce with other veterans. My grandfather was a gentle man with an awesome, Yoda-like wisdom, but he could also command a room.

In August 1972, years before I was born, Grandpa Shep had a massive stroke that left him with paralysis on his left side. But he didn't let this slow him down one bit. He still washed his dishes, got dressed, made his bed. And he was *extremely* neat and meticulous. Everything was pressed: sheets, clothes, you name it. When he came to live with us in 1996 (he and Grandma Shep had divorced a few years earlier), he had a few more comorbidities, including diabetes. I was twelve when I started helping him with his insulin—he took a fast-acting version of the hormone and a slow-acting one (I thought of them as "clear" and "cloudy") that needed to be mixed before being administered together. Can you imagine a twelve-year-old mixing insulin? Insulin is considered a "high-alert medication," as there is a heightened risk of significant patient harm when it is used in error. But I was diligent, cautious to a fault, and my mother always watched me to ensure I was pulling up the correct dose. My first caregiving experience was thus with someone whom I loved and cherished deeply. It made me realize healthcare was my path.

THREE YEARS LATER, when I was fifteen/sixteen, Grandma Shep's cousin died (yup, we were close with relatives that far removed). The funeral was at 10 a.m., but Grandpa Shep wasn't feeling well, so he decided to stay back. When my parents and I got back home after the service, we knew something was wrong as soon as we saw him. His speech was jumbled, he could barely move, and his face was drooping. I remember the trip to the emergency department like it was yesterday. It was obvious Grandpa Shep was having another stroke, but when we said this to the triage nurses, they seemed irritated and dismissed us with short, impatient answers. One of them told us we would have to stay in the waiting room with him and that he had to "wait to be seen like everyone else." I had no experience with hospitals at that point. My insulin-injecting job notwithstanding, I was still just a kid. But it didn't matter: it was clear that we were all, Grandpa Shep included, being treated horribly. We watched as patient after patient, none of whom looked as ill as Grandpa Shep, went in before him. It was only when patients who had arrived *after* us started going in that my mom finally decided she'd seen enough. I had never seen her that angry—she shouted at the nurses and demanded that my grandfather be seen. It was hard to shake the feeling that we were being treated differently, that the care we were receiving was subpar, unequal. And knowing what I know today, I can say definitively that it was.

While our diagnosis turned out, of course, to be the correct one, we did not anticipate the scope of it. Grandpa Shep experienced more than ten major strokes that day. He went into that hospital and never came out. I was in grade 9 during the eight months he spent in palliative care, and I would go to see him after school. Sometimes I'd even skip classes so I could feed him and help him get changed. I wiped food off his face, changed his linens, emptied his urinal. He'd always been fastidious—clean shaven, well-spoken—so it was devastating to see him in that unkempt, inarticulate state. A shell of himself. I remember two things clearly about that time: how difficult it was for my parents to navigate the healthcare system, and my growing awareness that I, a fifteen-year-old who had just started high school, was doing a better job caring for my grandfather than the nurses who were assigned to him.

Of the four patients in Grandpa Shep's room, he was the last to go. The fact that he outlived them might sound like a good thing, but the extra time also meant that we got to know and connect with his roommates and their families. And each individual loss felt like a punch in the gut.

Grandpa Shep passed away on October 7, 2001, just a day before his eighty-eighth birthday. We'd been expecting his death, of course, and yet I still didn't feel prepared for the emotion it unleashed in me. Grandma Shep came up from Florida for the funeral service, where she spoke warmly of him as the only man she had ever truly loved. There were over 200 people in attendance—family, friends, members of his Legion. It was truly a celebration of life. People told stories and shared experiences. They talked about the impact Grandpa had had on their lives. They remembered his infectious laugh and his handshake, which could shatter your forearm. Some stories were heartfelt and touching, others funny. We laughed and cried and finished with a traditional rendition of "It Is Well with My Soul."

But Grandpa Shep's passing didn't sit well with me. I couldn't imagine how I would ever fill the gaping hole it left in my soul. And it wasn't just me; we all felt his devastating loss profoundly.

Grandpa Shep's stroke and its aftermath was my first real exposure to the healthcare system. It was a brutal one. Decades later, I still get upset thinking about it. And the truth is that the system that created the inequities and disparities in healthcare outcomes hasn't changed much. I'm now well aware of how much more could have been done during Grandpa's intake and his time in hospital. His death might have been inevitable. What was lacking in the time leading up to it was the *care* that's in the very word *healthcare*.

MOTIVATED BY A general but somewhat unfocused desire to help people, after high school I enrolled in the Child and Youth Worker Program at Humber College in Toronto. It took a single semester to know that it wasn't where I wanted to be. I wanted to make the switch to nursing, but I didn't have the necessary prerequisites. Luckily, Humber had a one-year general arts and science program to help students bridge into a nursing or paramedic program. As soon as I heard about it, I eagerly enrolled.

At the end of my bridge year, however, the school suddenly pivoted and said that I, and several others who were attempting to do the same thing, wasn't eligible for the program I was applying for. I had crazy good grades—in chemistry, math, and physics my average was over 80 percent. I was furious.

Cue future speaker-advocate Amie. I called a big meeting with various stakeholders, including twelve other students who were in the same position I was—even my mom attended—and we proceeded to plead our case. We showed the school the information from its own website, which made it *abundantly* clear that students who enrolled in the General Arts and Science Technology Program could bridge into the Nursing Program. False advertising, we proclaimed. Many of us would have taken a different path had it not been for the promises the school made to us.

And guess what? Our protest worked! The school back-pedalled and kept its promise. We would all be allowed to bridge. It was a huge relief, especially since I'd been accepted into a four-year nursing program offered jointly by Humber College and the University of New Brunswick.

THE IDEA OF residence was actually scary to me, so in my first year I lived with my parents. Despite being outspoken and gregarious, I wasn't interested in that type of social scene. I was a homebody. But my parents had moved to a new subdivision and my commute, especially in winter, was a beast. Shelters weren't exactly all the rage in Brampton, and the transit itself was a nightmare. Luckily, I had met a special someone—my future husband, Jordan Varley—who lessened the pain of my commute with his awesomely stylish '91 Honda Civic.

It was 2006 and I was in my third year of nursing when Mom and I were in a bad car accident. We were approaching a light and I was in the passenger seat, bending over to pick up something that had fallen off my lap, when we were rear-ended by a Pontiac Grand Prix.

I blacked out. When I woke up, I was on the curb with a concussion and whiplash. I can't remember my reasoning, which obviously wasn't logical, but when the ambulance arrived I kept refusing to be taken to hospital. Mom also had whiplash, plus severe injuries to her hand and wrist. We both ended up doing five years of physio.

The accident shook me up and made me afraid to drive for a long time afterwards. Rehabilitation was slow, and my physical issues persisted. One of these was kidney damage, for which I needed multiple cystoscopies, a procedure that involves inserting a small telescope, called a ureteroscope, through the urethra and up into the bladder. When men have this procedure, a flexible tube is used, but with women it's an inflexible one, which, as you can imagine, is extremely painful. Nonsensical inequalities like this are part of the reason advocating for women's health has become so important to me.

I slowly got to the point where I felt ready to return to school. You'd think a nursing program would be able to offer accommodations for people with disabilities (I had a temporary one, plus chronic pain). But this one did not. The directors claimed they couldn't find a clinical placement that didn't involve standing for a long time, which at that point was really difficult for me. They offered no solutions or opportunities. I felt hurt, as well as disappointed by the apparent ableism of my chosen profession. With no leverage to get what I needed, I decided to leave nursing school until I got better.

PHYSICAL CHALLENGES ASIDE, my mind was still intact and eager for stimulation, so I enrolled in a biological and socio-cultural anthropology program at the University of Toronto. Most of my courses were at the university's Mississauga campus, so getting there involved really long bus rides. But I didn't mind. The campus and surrounding areas were beautiful. And I especially loved the forensic anthropology fieldwork that I did in years 2 and 3. I loved it so much, in fact, that at one point I considered becoming a forensic anthropologist (I've always harboured a not-so-secret passion for true crime). But then I discovered that there are only, like, two forensic anthropologists in all of Canada. I also learned that most forensics here are done by police, and it was a "hells to the no" about becoming a police officer! Back then they were talking about piloting civilians to do the work, but it wasn't a sure thing. I decided to stick with Plan A: nursing.

The things I learned about in my anthropology courses—human cultures, societies and evolution, and the rich histories of Indigenous Peoples—fascinated and grounded me. It was stuff that was never touched on in high school, and certainly not in nursing school. During those three years, it felt as if my brain was developing in a different way. Part of it was the fact that I was older, more mature, but I was aware of making intellectual connections that I hadn't made before. The process was exhilarating and eye-opening. I've maintained ever since that all nurses can benefit from studying socio-cultural anthropology. If our job is to treat human beings, to know their innermost workings, shouldn't we know about our evolution, culture, and diversity as a species?

I was now twenty-four years old, and because of my three-year break, I was officially in year eight of my four-year nursing degree. I knew that after year ten they kick you out, so I reached out to two of my professors, Kathleen White-Williams and Audrey Taves, for advice about re-entering the program. Honestly, I was scared about going back, but they reassured me that there was a place in nursing for someone like me and encouraged me to follow my heart. Thanks to their help, I succeeded and blew my fourth year out of the water.

MY FINAL YEAR, in most ways, was a breeze. I was thrilled to discover that the knowledge I'd acquired about anthropology was complementary to my nursing studies. I picked up some credits in Indigenous history, a subject that had taken on new resonance for me. The theoretical underpinnings of understanding culture, diversity, and different ways of knowing and being helped too. The icing on the cake was the solid investigative skills I'd acquired from my forensic anthropology fieldwork.

Having a high GPA meant that I could do clinical practicums in specialty areas that others didn't have access to, like obstetrics. Going in, I thought I knew what to expect, but my first experiences in labour and delivery were terrifying: the smell of blood, the family dynamics, and the whole "delivery" part. Later that year I did my consolidation at a hospital near to my home, and in June 2010 my degree was conferred. Despite those overwhelming early experiences in labour and delivery, I grew to love it—I still do—so when I got my first job in the specialty at the same hospital shortly after graduating, it felt fantastic.

IN 2011, I was pregnant with twins and preparing to go on maternity leave. I'd been, in my humble opinion, an exceptional labour and delivery nurse, and I assumed that that experience would help me navigate my own pregnancy and childbirth. But I don't think anything could have prepared me for what was to come. The hospital where I worked was classified as a Level 2C, meaning we dealt with uncomplicated births after 30 weeks. Any woman with an earlier gestation or a maternal/ fetal complication was sent to a specialty hospital (Level 3) like Mount Sinai in Toronto. As it turned out, none of the pregnancies or births I was involved with as a nurse was as complex as mine.

I'd heard the stats about higher morbidity and mortality rates, as well as premature births, among Black women, but none of it rang true until those numbers were particularized into *my* experience. The problems started before I even got pregnant. I had trouble with fertility due to a condition called polycystic ovary syndrome (PCOS). Having PCOS means, in a nutshell, that your body doesn't produce enough hormones to release an egg. Jordan and I tried to conceive for two years before we decided to go in for fertility treatment. People often talk about fertility treatments like it's some casual thing. It's not. There are the daily blood draws. The ultrasounds every three days to see what's happening in your cycle. Having to have sex every other day (daily is sometimes recommended) for ten days, which might sound fun, but I assure you isn't. Anxiety, coupled with performance issues, make this kind of sex dry, underwhelming, and very stressful. In contrast, when Jordan got tested for his fertility, he was sent to the bathroom with a porn mag. So yeah, the experience is pretty darn different for women than for men.

They put me on Clomid, a medication that helps you produce more eggs. Amazingly, it worked. I got pregnant almost right away (three cycles later). But when they tested the level of my HCG (the hormone that indicates how far along you are), the numbers kept tripling. We were having twins!! Jordan and I were overjoyed.

When I was around 14 or 15 weeks pregnant, my blood pressure started creeping up. I felt fine, but of course you don't *feel* high blood pressure, which is why they call it the silent killer. The signs that I was getting pre-eclampsia were becoming too obvious to ignore. So far, I had been in the care of a high-risk specialist I'd worked with in Brampton. Dr. Persad now wanted me to consult with Dr. Barrett, a maternal fetal specialist who'd done research on Black women's morbidity and mortality and was one of the country's most renowned specialists on twins. I felt fortunate to be in the care of these two amazing, top-notch doctors.

But after 21 weeks, Dr. Persad announced that she wasn't able to treat me anymore due to the increased complexity of my pregnancy and growing concerns of pre-eclampsia. My blood pressure was completely out of control, and with a risk of going into early labour, I would now be solely under Dr. Barrett's care. At 28 weeks, I was admitted to Sunnybrook, a major-trauma hospital northeast of Toronto, where, in one of my daily ultrasounds, I was found to have intrauterine growth restriction. This meant that one twin wasn't growing as fast as the other. This twin was also experiencing placental insufficiency, a situation that can lead to neurological issues after birth. On top of all this, I was showing signs of eclampsia and high liver enzymes, which put me at risk of seizures and maternal or infant death. The joy Jordan and I had felt when we finally learned I was pregnant seemed like a thing of the distant past. All I felt now was fear.

I'd been at Sunnybrook for three weeks on the morning I woke up with contractions. A full-term pregnancy is 40 weeks, and I was at 31 weeks, 2 days. I'd never experienced such pain. Dr. Barrett was away, so Dr. Cohen stepped in and delivered the twins by C-section with a staff of at least twenty, all of whom were actively participating in the delivery. There were two teams, one for each baby. Twin A, Tristan, came first. Even though he weighed a reasonably healthy four pounds, he was immediately whisked away to the Neonatal Intensive Care Unit. Things were happening fast, and it was scary. Two minutes later Twin B, Logan, was born at a mere two pounds.

During the first birth, I remember feeling pressure, then nothing. I blacked out before the second birth. Concerned that I would have more complications after delivery, staff kept me in for observation for two more days. Then I was discharged, but the twins had to stay. Brampton, where we lived, is basically on the opposite side of Toronto from Sunnybrook, so getting to see them took two hours. It was painful that they were so far away, but I made it a point to spend up to eight hours, sometimes more, at their side.

And my troubles weren't over yet. On the first night after I got home, I started having trouble breathing. Just walking from the living room to the kitchen winded me. My legs were so swollen they looked like tree trunks. My nursing experience hadn't proved very useful with my pregnancy, but this time I knew exactly what I was dealing with. I turned to Jordan and said, "I think I have a pulmonary embolism."

I called Dr. Persad, who told me to get to the hospital immediately. Minutes later we were in the car, heading to emerg at Brampton Civic Hospital, a 20-minute drive away. When we arrived, Jordan explained to the triage nurse how sick I was. She looked at my exhausted husband—normally well groomed, he now had a thick beard and long, scraggly hair from weeks of living at Sunnybrook Hospital—and motioned him (and me) to sit down. He told her I might die, to which she responded sarcastically that *she* might die if she didn't go on break soon.

Now Jordan is the most kind, gentle-hearted person you'll ever meet. But at this point he lost his shit. "You need to do your fucking job!" he yelled. (Despite my discomfort and panic, I was still shocked when he did this.)

Just as that interaction was occurring, Dr. Persad came down and expeditiously made arrangements to get me to the cardio-respirology unit. I was admitted in short order and diagnosed with congestive heart failure, pulmonary edema, and—you guessed it—a pulmonary embolism. In the moment, I was scared that I too would end up just another statistic about Black patients in healthcare. Like Grandpa Shep. Or like Grandma Shep, who would die in my mom's arms from a massive pulmonary embolism six months later, mere steps from the Florida hospital unit from which she'd just been discharged.

In the respirology unit, while pumping milk and tethered to a million beeping monitors, I begged Jordan to go be with the twins. But he was torn. He'd been so afraid of losing them after they were born. Now he was afraid of losing me as well; we both knew that dying wasn't an uncommon outcome of pre-eclampsia. What we didn't yet know was that, although delivering a baby massively reduces symptoms of pre-eclampsia, a deadly postpartum form of the condition can persist. This was what I had. All the symptoms I'd experienced before birth—difficulty breathing, rapid heart rate, elevated liver enzymes—were signs that my body was shutting down, and the symptoms were now worse.

The week I spent at Brampton Civic was torture. I kept thinking about my babies, so tiny and far away in their incubators. At one point I couldn't take it anymore and asked hospital staff to let me leave to go see my children. They denied the request, which was the right thing to do, so I decided to take matters into my own hands and snuck out. They weren't happy about this—technically I would qualify as a Code Yellow or "missing patient"—but I think deep down some of them understood, and probably would have done the same thing in my position.

After a month at Sunnybrook, the boys were moved to Brampton Hospital. Having them so much closer to home was a huge relief. And while I slowly got better, the question kept hanging over me: would I have ended up another faceless statistic had I not gone to the hospital when I did? According to a recent article in *Chatelaine* magazine, Canada has a "dearth of race-based data within our public institutions, an issue that stems in part from a general hesitancy to talk about race and racism in this country." But we can't ignore the statistics in the US and the UK, where, according to the same article, Black women have the most pregnancy-related deaths of any demographic.

I WENT BACK to work in labour and delivery a year after the twins were born. I assumed all my health scares were now behind me, and that my new life as a mom would settle into an easy rhythm. This assumption proved misplaced. Following up on the twins' care was complex and involved endless health appointments. Then in 2013, at two years old, Tristan (Twin A) was diagnosed with autism. A few years later, Logan (Twin B) was diagnosed with ADHD. I admit I struggled with these things. After everything I'd been through trying to conceive, the difficult pregnancy and birth, almost dying of postpartum pre-eclampsia, and dealing with medically complex twins, was it too much to ask for children who were just . . . healthy?

But, of course, life doesn't work that way. It's not a series of rewards and punishments that balance out. You get what you get, and what I got was a shiny new role as a mom of two children with disabilities. It was an isolating time. Jordan was working in Cold Lake, Alberta, as a manager in the oil patch. When the twins were about six months old, we went out to join him, but his work was an eight-hour drive from where we lived, in Cochrane. This meant we didn't see him all that often, and so my loneliness persisted.

Intending to fight it, and to embrace the west, I took on some part-time nursing teaching. But after a year it had become clear that this was not the place for me. I was struggling with postpartum depression and had flown my mom and dad out several times so they could support me. After some long conversations, Jordan and I mutually decided that it would be best for me to return home to Brampton. He would travel back and forth to visit me and the kids whenever he could.

A few months after I got back to Ontario, I started feeling unwell. To my great surprise and joy, I discovered I was pregnant. Fourteen weeks in, however, I woke up in excruciating pain and was taken by ambulance to emerg. The pregnancy was ectopic, meaning the fetus was growing outside my uterus, so I ended up losing it, along with my right fallopian tube. (In the US, since *Roe v. Wade* was overturned it is no longer standard procedure to end an ectopic pregnancy, and women are dying as a result.) It was devastating. We'd already told the family, made big plans, had hopes and dreams for this little one who was gone all too soon.

With two energetic boys at home and still reeling from loss, I knew I needed a change of pace in my professional life. Shift work was not a good fit for the challenges I was facing, so I started to look at going back to school. I had developed a bit of a taste for academia, and because I'd been lucky enough to secure a part-time faculty nursing position prior to having the boys, I felt I could do more teaching. I returned to U of T, this time to do my master's degree in clinical nursing with a specialty in women's health and collaborative nursing. And because hope springs eternal, I was pregnant again, this time with my daughter. I needed a break from the demands of bedside nursing and a master's would be just the ticket, making me eligible for a less frenetic leadership role.

MY FIRST LEADERSHIP position was as a part-time clinical nurse educator in the obstetrics ward of a hospital. Although I started the job full of hope, I wasn't prepared for the sheer amount of bureaucracy or the negative environment, and the disappointment set in almost immediately. (Looking back now, I think I had unrealistic expectations.)

The staff, on the other hand, were great. And one was Sara, who was working there as a clinical nurse specialist. Many of the others had been colleagues of mine during the two years I worked as a labour and emergency nurse, an adrenaline-fuelled role that requires sharp critical thinking skills and the ability to react quickly. So I guess you could say that when I returned in my nurse-educator capacity, I already had a certain street cred. We'd been in the trenches together. We'd bonded over labouring patients and shared gripes in the nursing lounge about the lack of staffing. Nurses tend to respect those with whom they've shared experiences, which is why this group in particular trusted me. In labour and delivery, nurses are like a wolf pack; if you're not part of it, they'll eat you alive.

Unfortunately, Sara was not seen as part of that pack. Though I saw her mostly in passing, it was clear she was having trouble being accepted by the other nurses, who viewed her as an outsider. In the end, it was going on mat leave that gave her a way out.

OUR PATHS CROSSED next at another hospital where I had accepted a full-time position in the maternal-child program. About a year into the job, I learned that they were looking for a professional practice clinician in pediatrics, specifically the NICU, and I immediately thought of Sara. I knew she had experience in the field and didn't want to go back to her previous employer due to her negative experiences with staff there. So although she was still on mat leave at the time, I encouraged her to apply.

She got the job, and we ended up sharing an office. The space was tight but homey, with a single frosted-glass window that, when the sun hit just right, warmed everything up. I showed her the ropes, and we quickly bonded through our many shared interests: children's clothing, Thai brunches, and being nurses in new leadership roles. Sara made sure that I went to the bathroom, sometimes pushing me there on my rolly chair (I know this probably sounds strange, but not going to the bathroom is a chronic problem if you're a nurse. We get so busy we forget!)

I couldn't have asked for a better group of nurses to work with in that maternal-child program. Although I wasn't on the front lines myself, I showed up for them. They would come to me with their personal and professional concerns, whether it was a question about their kids, a policy that needed reviewing, or a practice that needed to be implemented, or maybe they just needed a shoulder to cry on. I'd do whatever was in my power to mobilize change and make sure they felt supported. We were all passionate about what we were doing.

But the honeymoon phase didn't last. My workload quickly went from manageable to unmanageable due to the administration's completely unrealistic expectations. Every day, I felt like I was being told to dig six one-foot-deep holes instead of one six-foot-deep hole. And I did not yet have the advocacy skills to stand up for myself, as I do now.

One of the hardest parts of leadership nursing is the endless meetings. And after they're done you still have to do the work, helping nurses with educational requirements, simulation exercises, new-hire training, hands-on support, etc. Even worse: because you never have enough time to dedicate yourself fully to one thing, you end up pleasing no one. It can get really frustrating. It's also something that nurses who aren't in a leadership role sometimes have trouble understanding.

Another major issue was the disconnect between what our nurses needed and what the administration wanted. I knew what being on the front lines felt like, but the leadership above me didn't.

But the biggest problem of all was that I began to experience bullying, gaslighting, and harassment. A typical example: We would call a meeting with administrators and educators to deal with a situation. We'd reach an agreement. Then, at a larger team meeting with obstetricians and other healthcare professionals, one administrator would pretend we hadn't come to that agreement. I forwarded email exchanges and notes I'd taken during the meeting, but she still denied what I knew to be reality. This administrator belittled me and made me feel stupid and crazy. I couldn't believe the harassment and disrespect that was taking place. (What's crazy is that Sara and I were essentially having the same experiences, but we didn't talk about them. I think we both knew it was happening to the other, but our mutual fear kept us silent.)

All the time I was working there, the administrator pretended she was an open door, asking us to come to her with ideas, but I quickly realized this was BS. When someone did present her with an idea or offer a suggestion, she often tried to take credit for it. The gaslighting began the day she contradicted me in public, yelling at me like I was nothing. Colleagues who witnessed one of these interactions would pull me aside to tell me how wrong it was, how she never spoke like that to anyone but me. Still, it took a while before I summoned the courage to ask to meet with the administrator privately. I wanted to talk about what had happened (or at the very least convince myself I wasn't going crazy). At that meeting, she surprised me by admitting that she had been wrong. She had yelled at me and treated me badly, she said, because I wasn't taking her direction. In other words, it was a dominance play. Without saying so directly, she was also admitting that I intimidated her. The open-door, open-opinion environment she claimed to be nurturing was all a lie.

At the same time, I was constantly being asked to do unethical things that weren't part of my job description, like observe night-shift nurses and suggest staff cuts that would help solve budget problems. The administrator wanted me to figure out a fiscal workaround that would make her look good. But budgets were her area, not mine. My job was to practise evidence-based nursing, ensure the safety of patients and their families, and get nurses the resources they needed. It wasn't to get people laid off. What she asked made me deeply uncomfortable, but I was too terrified of her to be openly defiant. Instead, I asked if the request benchmarked with other hospitals, to which I was told that we just had to "find a way to do it."

In April 2018, my mom called me at work and told me she was having another episode of supraventricular tachycardia, a condition in which your heart's electrical signals misfire, resulting in an irregularly fast or erratic heart rate (arrhythmia) even when you're sitting still. I knew the situation was life threatening—she could die if they didn't cardiovert her fast enough—so she asked if I could meet her downstairs in the emergency department. Even though I knew I had to go, I still felt nervous, imagining how the administrator would respond.

I told my mother I'd visit her during my lunch hour, but that I'd have to go back to work as soon as it was over. I messaged the administrator to let her know my mom was in hospital, and that I was going to use my own time to see her. When I got no response, I went about my business until lunch. When I got to emerg, Mom was being set up for EKG bloodwork and telemetry. There was a decent risk she would have a cardiac event right there in the hospital. She looked ill, and I felt worried. Before I left, I kissed her and told her I'd be down again right after work. I also called Jordan and asked him to follow up with her as soon as he could. Leaving felt gut-wrenching.

I took the elevator up to my office and was back at my desk right on time. I was sweating bullets from the dual stress of my mom's illness and the possibility that I'd get grief about going to visit her. I couldn't believe that a rational fear for my mom's life was being overridden by an irrational fear of a negative interaction.

Back at work, I continued an email thread (on which the administrator was cc'ed) with an anaesthesiologist about a C-section project we'd all agreed to pause. Several emails from the administrator followed, then suddenly she was coming down the hall, her heels clacking even more loudly than usual. My anxiety went through the roof. She walked into the office with a smug, judgmental look and started peppering me with questions that she didn't allow me to answer, cutting me off each time. Her tone was condescending, tyrannical. She knew my mom was downstairs facing a life-threatening situation. It was clear that she simply didn't care.

This realization was the straw that broke the camel's back, or at least my brain. I had already been experiencing panic attacks at work that made me feel like I was going to die. Sometimes when I heard the administrator coming down the hall, I—a grown woman—would turn the lights off and hide under my desk. There were days when I was super depressed and cried at work. My doctor had upped my anti-anxiety meds, but it didn't really help. As things with the administrator escalated, I decided to keep a detailed log of all our interactions.

My blood pressure was going up at an alarming rate and I felt suicidal. My self-esteem, never an issue in the past, was eroding. Knowing the time had finally come to take my health seriously, I went to the Occupational Health department to request mental health leave. I explained that I was feeling stress that wasn't related to workload but to an individual who was targeting me and bullying me.

I knew I couldn't be the first employee to experience a problem like this. But I was astounded to learn that the department had no framework to deal with it, no systems of support. Everything in the occupational health forms was about "physical limitations," not psychological ones. They didn't know what to do with me.

I took two weeks of stress leave. But the bullying continued, even in my absence. Three days into my leave, the administrator sent an email to nursing staff and the entire mat-child team that very pointedly made mention of "resiliency."

I SHOULD HAVE stayed on leave longer. I wasn't well enough to go back, but I felt coerced to do so. The hospital sent a return-to-work plan that allowed me to work on a different unit temporarily, but with the longer-term goal being that I would return to the same unit, with the same administrator.

My return was predictably horrible. As I expected, nothing had been put in place to keep me safe from the administrator. After multiple conversations with HR, I finally got the opportunity to speak to her boss. But she ignored my explanations—even though I explicitly and repeatedly stated that my problems weren't with workload but with a single individual—and focused instead on work pressures.

"Maybe this isn't your time at this hospital," she had the nerve to say to me. WTF?

Cue, once again, future speaker-advocate Amie. I wrote a letter to the director of HR in which I described my situation and stated that the organization wasn't treating people with mental health stress appropriately. I spoke to the hospital's VP, who said she would follow up to ensure that what had happened to me would never happen again, to me or to anyone else. That was the last I heard from her. I kept up my complaints. An "investigation" was launched. Sara and I were both interviewed, but nothing ever came of that either. My case was at a dead end.

Sara went on mental health leave two weeks after I did. No one in Occupational Health or the administration seemed to view this strange coincidence as the symptom of a deeper problem, something requiring examination.

Sara and I were two of only five racialized nurses in leadership at that hospital. Everyone else was white, including the administration. I was often told by staff members who witnessed the micro- and macro-aggressions aimed at me that I was treated and spoken to differently than our other colleagues. After Sara and I took our leaves, they brought in a Black person to HR. It felt like a token move, like they were covering their asses. What I was dealing with had a name: racist abuse. I knew then that I could never go back to that maternal-child department.

THE ONE POSITIVE outcome of this was that Sara and I were finally talking openly to each other about the administrator. We asked ourselves: seeing that we had both undergone such horrible treatment, why was nothing done about it? The two of us had shared a lot of similar experiences during our nursing journeys, not all of them happy. But good things happened to both of us after we left that facility for other jobs. One was that, for the first time, each of us had a male boss that we really, really liked.

Another was the podcast. When I suggested the idea to Sara—including the title, *The Gritty Nurse Podcast*—she was immediately sold on it. The podcasting world felt like it was dominated by men, especially in the realms of science and medicine. In other words, it seemed like the perfect time for two racialized, resilient nurses to enter the room.

Nursing has always had a huge gender component. Although female physicians now outnumber their male colleagues, female nurses have traditionally been seen as "handmaidens" to male doctors, toiling along in their shadow. And the fact that almost all nurses were female meant that women were put in adversarial roles, competing against one another for a limited number of spots. We've both seen this play out all too many times.

Going into my new job with the Niagara Health hospital system, I had the powerful feeling that these were my people. Admittedly, it was a feeling I'd had before, one that usually went away after a year or so. I had been diagnosed with depression and anxiety, and was scared of being treated the same way as before. But I got lucky. Fred, my new boss, who had been a nurse himself, was 100 percent the person I needed at that delicate time in my life. He didn't know the full extent of my ordeal at my previous job, but he didn't need to. He was just . . . kind. I needed a manager who would encourage me to grow and to be myself, while also allowing some flexibility for my situation (having a child with a disability, changing and adjusting my anxiety meds, etc.). Fred did all of this.

If there was work to be done, Fred's default check-in was "Do you need support? Resources?" or "How can I help you succeed?" Then he'd give us the resources and say, "Okay, get it done!" He was that kind of boss. The good kind. At my previous job, I'd gotten used to non-stop micro-management. At Niagara Health, instead of going on mental health leave, we went to courses. Fred's frequent catchphrase, "It's a journey," reflected his gentle temperament. Fred retired a few years later, but I will never forget his leadership or his kindness, both of which had a huge positive impact on me at a crucial time in my life.

NURSE *WITH* GRIT

Harriet Tubman (1822–1913)

Everyone knows Harriet Tubman was a former slave and a conductor on the Underground Railroad, where she earned the moniker "Moses of Her People." Few are aware that she was also a nurse who cared for Black Union Army soldiers and liberated slaves during the Civil War. In 1908, she used property she had bought in Auburn, New York, to establish the Harriet Tubman Home for Aged and Indigent Negroes. Per Tubman's intention, the facility continued to care for the poor and elderly of the community well after her death in 1913. It's safe to say that Tubman could not have done the work she did without a nursing background, so let's get her official credential changed to "Underground Railroad conductor *and nurse*"!

Debi Wade

*I*t's a Wednesday morning, and RN Debi Wade is standing in front of the door of an apartment in St. Jamestown, a dense Toronto neighbourhood made up of high-rises where many low-income people live. She's come to see Lisa, a client she's never met before. All she knows about Lisa is that she's heavily pregnant with her first child and has an intellectual disability. But when Debi knocks, Lisa doesn't answer. Instead, a woman emerges from the apartment next door. It's Lisa's mother-in-law, and she helpfully unlocks Lisa's door for Debi.

The overwhelming stench that greets her when she walks in, along with the mountains of stuff everywhere, makes it abundantly clear that this is a hoarding situation. Debi squeezes through a narrow passageway through the mix of household debris and garbage and makes her way to the back of the apartment. She finds Lisa in bed but unresponsive and calls 911. Firefighters and EMS staff arrive shortly after, but getting Lisa out of the apartment is challenging given her condition and the state of the apartment. Lisa's mother-in-law comes out of her own apartment again but doesn't say anything or even seem curious about the drama unfolding in front of her. Debi is pretty sure she has an intellectual disability too.

Debi rides with her unconscious client in the ambulance to the hospital, where it's determined that Lisa has illegal drugs in her system. Debi will help Lisa with her substance abuse problems over the remaining weeks of her pregnancy, but it won't be enough. Lisa's baby is apprehended by the Children's Aid Society shortly after birth.

For Lisa, this is devastating. Despite her personal problems, and the fact that there's no father in the picture, she'd been excited about the prospect of having a child. Debi has a lot of empathy for Lisa. Although she pegs her at about a grade 2 level intellectually, she finds her agreeable and receptive. After the baby is gone, Debi helps Lisa deal with her postpartum bleeding and shows her how to stop the milk that's making her breasts painfully hard. She does a lot of listening. Lisa seems unable to entirely comprehend the situation and keeps asking when she'll get her baby back. In order for that to happen, Debi tells her, she needs to listen carefully to the CAS and show them that she's learned from her mistakes and can be a good parent in the future.

After these interactions, Debi's work with Lisa will be done. She is mandated to work only with families, not individuals, which Lisa now officially is. This could change if Lisa can show the CAS she's a responsible parent and gets her baby back, but for now, Debi closes the file.

IT'S BEEN HARD to find a nurse lately who hasn't considered leaving the profession. Forty-one-year-old Debi Wade isn't one of them. Debi loves her work as a public health nurse, which she's been doing for fifteen years. Her enthusiasm stems from the diversity of the work itself, the sense of connection and follow-through she gets with her clients, and the positive outcomes she helps bring about.

Like many nurses, Debi started at the bedside, taking a position in the NICU in 2004. Working with babies initially sounded like a great gig, but despite a six-month orientation the experience itself was frequently terrifying. She often had trouble sleeping the night before a shift, worrying about what she would face the next day. By 2006, in need of a break, she applied for and got a nursing position in New Zealand. It was also in the NICU, but she thought the change of locale might make the experience different. She was right. In New Zealand, she had even more responsibility. Her hospital only had nurses and doctors—there were no respiratory therapists, registered dietitians, or nurse practitioners—so Debi did tasks like pulling and spinning her patients' blood (something that, back home, was normally done at a lab), then analyzing the results to make decisions about ventilation changes. Over the year she spent in New Zealand, her growing experience and proficiency with an increasing number of skills boosted her confidence significantly.

It also gave her some perspective on her still-budding career, so that by the time she returned to Canada she was ready to try something new. A major factor was her strong aversion to night shifts. (Debi is someone who thrives on routine and getting to bed early.) Everything she heard about community health made her think it might suit her. Best of all, there were no night shifts! When she applied for a job in the field she got no response, so she enrolled in a master's program in public health, only to drop out a few months later. The classes felt overwhelming, and she concluded that she just wasn't ready to go back to school.

Debi was feeling down on herself and unsure what to do next when, out of the blue, she was offered a position in, of all things, public health. It all felt a bit like serendipity.

After the high-stakes tension of working in the NICU, Debi figured community health would be a cakewalk, but it turned out to be challenging in a different way. First, there was the element of surprise. When she was sent to a client's home for the first time, she usually had no idea what would be waiting for her on the other side of the door. And she soon realized that to succeed as a public health nurse she needed to gain the trust of her clients. To do this, she required better soft skills, especially in communication.

This was no small thing. As a child, Debi was so shy and reserved that she didn't even like to smile (this is definitely not the case now). When she first started in NICU, speaking to parents made her incredibly nervous. This gradually changed over time as she gained skills and self-assurance. The fact that making connections with her patients is what she loves best about her work these days—and what's more, that she's really *good* at it—surprises her more than anyone. She credits nursing with bringing her out of her shell, making her easier and more open with people.

Nursing might seem a strange choice for someone so timid, but Debi started dealing with the healthcare system at a relatively early age. When she was twelve, her dad had a kidney transplant and was frequently in and out of hospitals. He *loved* the nurses, and this admiration strongly influenced her decision to go into the profession. (Oddly enough, kidney transplants have been a bit of a thing in her life. Two kids in her grade 10 class had them; one was her future husband.)

Debi met Lisa in 2007 while working at her first public health job with Ontario's Healthy Babies Healthy Children program. The program was open to women with risk factors ranging from low incomes to traumatic birth. Debi's main task was to help disadvantaged women pre- and postpartum. Like all public health programs, its goals were preventative. The goal was to help families in the community so that their babies didn't end up in the hospital or the NICU.

Seven years later, she took a public health position on a pilot project called Investing in Families, which was run through the Ontario Works Assistance program. The aim of the project was to give families who had an unemployed member the necessary support to get the member working again. Many of Debi's clients lived in the Jane and Finch area, a notorious, at times unfairly maligned Toronto neighbourhood of dense high-rises known for its low-income demographics and high crime rates.

One of the things that surprised Debi about her new job was the intimacy. The women she met in the Healthy Babies Healthy Children program told her things they wouldn't tell their mothers or their best friends—their fears around becoming a new mom or the sadness they sometimes experienced. Her clients asked Debi questions they didn't ask other people because they were afraid to appear "stupid." Many were newcomers to the country who lacked basic English skills. Some suffered from postpartum depression and anxiety and were convinced something was wrong with their child (Debi's own experience with postpartum depression helped her better understand what these women were going through); others needed more specialized psychiatric treatment. But Debi saw that many simply lacked confidence. She found she could empower these clients simply through reassurance and information.

Debi had grown up relatively sheltered in a middle-class Toronto suburb, so much of what she initially saw in community health was eye-opening, if not shocking. At times she had trouble taking it all in.

She remembers going to see a family of new immigrants from China at what she took to be their house. But after being greeted at the front door, she was led down to the basement and up some dank stairs to what amounted to a shed in the backyard. It had no bathroom, and the only source of heat was a small electric space heater. The clients were essentially living in pioneer conditions in the middle of a major Canadian city in winter. The family would become one of Debi's early success stories when she eventually helped to set them up in a warm basement apartment in Scarborough, a suburb in the east end of the city.

Another of her early clients was Maria, a mom in her late twenties. She had fled from her abusive husband in Mexico by pretending she was taking their son to school, going straight to the airport and taking a plane to Toronto. They arrived with no English and no connections. All Maria knew about her new country was what she had learned from basic googling. She and her son had left everything behind in Mexico, including the beloved family dog.

Debi got Maria set up with a family doctor and mental health supports and connected her with the city's substantial Spanish-speaking population. She enrolled her son at the local school, where the grade 2 teacher spoke Spanish, and registered him with the City's recreation department so he could access sports and other extra-curricular activities. To address some of his behavioural issues, she enlisted the help of the Child Development Institute. As a way of getting to know her adopted city, Maria expressed a desire to volunteer, so Debi lined up a variety of options for her. It meant everything to Debi when Maria told her, "You're proving to me I was right in coming here."

When she started in community health, Debi didn't understand how she could possibly make a difference in her clients' lives, which often seemed so desperate. But as time went by, she began to see how doing what seemed like small things could make a difference. One client, Luz, had two sons, a seventeen-year-old and a fourteen-year-old who was severely autistic. Luz had reluctantly come to the realization that her younger son needed to live in a group home. The older boy had to care for his brother when she went to work in a grocery store, and it was an unsustainable situation for everyone. Debi wrote down the steps that were necessary to apply to the group home and helped Luz organize all her documents. She got Luz's son on the wait list of the Pathways program with the expectation he would be accepted the following spring.

One of the cases Debi is most proud of is that of Juanita, a single mother from Mexico. Juanita had two daughters, a twelve-year-old and a four-year-old. The elder had cerebral palsy and used a wheelchair. She was nonverbal and ate through a feeding tube. Overwhelmed and exhausted, Juanita was so consumed with caring for this child—she was often up all night long—that her four-year-old was for all intents and purposes forgotten: she, too, was nonverbal and not yet toilet trained. She wasn't enrolled in kindergarten, so Debi did this right away. Within weeks, she also had her toilet trained. She checked in regularly with the kindergarten teacher and arranged for an educational assessment and diagnosis. By the time she closed the family's case in March 2020, things had improved significantly. The younger girl was well supported in grade 1. She loved school, could speak and understand English, and had several close friends, so her social skills were growing rapidly. A PSW came daily to do activities with the older child, giving Juanita some needed respite. One of the things that had been holding Juanita back was her lack of English, so Debi got her enrolled in online classes. When Debi left her, Juanita was full of hope and planning to find a full-time job in the near future.

Another client, Beverly, had come on her own from the Caribbean as a teenager to escape a bad family situation. When Debi met Beverly, she was living as a single parent in a two-bedroom apartment and had four kids. Two were in school, and the other two were in the NICU at SickKids hospital. Debi supported Beverly's children for the four months they were in the NICU through to their discharge. Beverly's personal goal was to find work; to help make that happen, Debi got her on a child-care subsidy waiting list. It took three years, but she eventually got the spot and, shortly after, a job at Winners. Beverly's children were from three different fathers, and she had a rocky relationship with each of them, so Debi served as Beverly's advocate as she navigated legal processes around custody. She even attended court with her, providing emotional support by reminding Beverly how far she had come.

You might be reading all this and thinking, "Hold on, isn't this . . . *social work?*" Debi is aware of the similarities, but she points to the fact that there are no social workers in public health, so the nursing skill set often comes closest to filling those needs. A lot of Debi's job involves answering her clients' health-related questions, teaching them to navigate the healthcare system, and filling out a ton of paperwork, but she likes the variety. "Nursing is a lot more than people think. Even my in-laws were surprised," she says.

Debi has come to see her role as helping her clients build resiliency. Accomplishing this evokes that famous saying: if you give someone a fish you feed them for a day, but if you teach them to fish you feed them for a lifetime. Sometimes "support" means listening to a client as they unburden themselves of their life story. Other times it means empowering them with good information.

Her workplace is anywhere and everywhere. Sometimes the client will come to her office, which she encourages, especially if it's a female client and Debi suspects there's abuse going on at home. If this is the case—and sadly, it's not rare—she'll come up with a safety plan for if and when the woman wants to go to a shelter.

Other times she'll meet the client at their home, or in a public library. Maya wanted Debi to come to the high-rise apartment complex where she'd lived since she was eleven years old so she could witness first-hand the way she was being harassed by another resident. Someone was intentionally dropping dirty diapers and other objects outside her ground-floor window. She also thought she and her children were being followed. Maya could handle herself, but she worried about her children walking to school, which was directly across from and facing her building. Debi arranged for the school vice-principal to personally receive the children when they arrived in the morning. She also enrolled them in MLSE LaunchPad, a sports program for underserved communities. Knowing that others in the community cared about and had eyes on her children was important to Maya, not to mention a huge relief.

Debi had ninety families on her roster until March 2020, when she was suddenly cut off from all of them after the Investing in Families program shut down its nursing component in reaction to the pandemic. It was a wrenching time for Debi and her clients. Some continued to call her, looking for support with their kids' schooling or special needs meetings, or for their mental health. One family had a child who needed back surgery, and the mom, who lacked English skills, kept calling to request Debi's help in the hospital and discharge meetings, where she often found herself confused.

Over the course of the next two and a half years, Debi was redeployed into ten other positions, including providing support at a shelter and administering vaccines at a clinic. After her experience at the latter, she wrote an official procedure for vaccinating children under twelve without their parents present. The Covid whirlwind was exhausting, but Debi says it helped round out her skills and gave her a handle on what it takes to be a great community health nurse. The Investing in Families program was relaunched in July 2022, and Debi and a few other nurses were re-recruited to get things up to speed again, albeit with a much-reduced number of clients. Debi's manager praised her work and told her she seemed like an entirely different person, which she took as the compliment it was intended to be.

DEBI HAS LEARNED to compartmentalize her work—a necessary skill in healthcare. But every once in a while, when she describes her day to her husband, the appalled look on his face reminds her that what she deals with on a daily basis isn't, or shouldn't be, normal.

Compartmentalizing doesn't mean being immune or insensitive to patients' pain, however. Debi still gets down some days, especially when it comes to kids, many of whom live in depressing surroundings with mice running around and the TV on all day. She visits children who eat nothing but pasta, or junk food, and aren't going to school because their parents can't afford to accompany them on public transit. She takes all these issues on as best as she can, by helping parents with budgeting, teaching them how to read nutrition labels, or locating food banks. Since public health is about disease prevention, Debi knows that the healthier they eat, the healthier they'll be. And while she also knows that the public programs her clients employ can make a real difference in their lives, the paltry amount of government welfare many are forced to live on strikes her as deeply unfair.

Treating their mental health issues is often key to getting her clients on their feet. Debi will get them enrolled in the free programs first, usually group therapy. Once they have an income, she will help them find a therapist who charges fees on a sliding scale. Some people initially resist therapy, which they may see as stigmatizing, but she encourages them to try it, knowing it can make a big difference right away. She's become familiar with the signs of improvement: A client will show up for their meeting *not* wearing pyjamas. They'll exhibit energy and optimism or talk about their kids in a positive way. As for the kids themselves, Debi sees regular school attendance as the sign that things are turning around for them.

"Someone once asked me, Don't you get mad at your clients? And I always say no. Their lives are so hard, I'm not surprised they're not working. Many have mental health struggles and can't get up in the morning. They're in survival mode. I'm there to help them break down the problems and provide support where they need it in order to reach whatever goals they have. I can never judge anyone because I don't know what it's like to live their day to day."

Public health is one of the few areas of nursing where there's patient continuity. Nurses in labour and delivery, medical surgical (med-surg), NICU, or postpartum—to name just a few—rarely see their patients again after they're discharged, except by happenstance. Part of what keeps Debi interested in and passionate about her work is seeing that she's making people's lives better. She feels that her job allows her to grow personally and professionally. With the exodus from nursing, it seems there's a lesson here for the profession as a whole. Would more bedside nurses stick around if they enjoyed the same feeling of satisfaction in accomplishment?

Debi will never go back to bedside nursing full-time, but she thinks it's important to keep a foot in clinical practice, so she also works part-time, maybe once a week, at a Toronto NICU. Her hospital is a Level 2, which means the babies are often intubated or on oxygen support, but the expectation is that they'll get better, and the end goal is to bring them home. On a typical shift Debi will care for maybe three or four infants—feeding and changing them, giving them their meds, checking their vitals, and calling for help when something goes wrong. But her favourite part of the job is prepping and educating families for the transition home. As in her community health work, she encourages anxious parents to be hands-on, to change the child's diaper or just to hold them. And she helps them navigate the healthcare system. After the doctor comes by on rounds, parents often turn to Debi with a bewildered look and ask, "What just happened?" As the seasoned, skilled, confident professional she is, she's only too happy to explain.

THE TUNNEL (A GHOST STORY)

Sara

Every nurse knows a ghost story, even if they're not always willing to share it with outsiders. Ours is a science-based profession, so it's not surprising that some of us are worried about appearing irrational or superstitious. We spend a lot of time with death. When you become a hospital nurse you operate on the assumption that someone has died in every bed. It's not creepy, it's just a reality of the job.

And yet things have happened, to us and to many others we know, that we've struggled to explain. Often, they become part of our private folklore. Most of the spirits—if I can call them that—we encounter don't seem evil. Like, for instance, the gentleman in Room 221 of a certain hospital, who used to yank the sheets off nurses who were having a nap in that room (like he did to his own bedcovers when he was a patient and his body temperature was high). But then there are those hospital rooms where things always seem to go south. Rooms that feel, to use a very unscientific term, cursed. None of us wants to believe this is true, but it's a hard feeling to shake.

ONE OF THE freakiest things that ever happened to me on the job occurred on the tenth floor of a downtown Toronto hospital. It was around 7 a.m. on a Sunday. I'd just finished working the night shift in postpartum and was wearily making my way to the elevator bank. There was no one around. It felt like I had the entire floor to myself. People who are used to the bustle of a hospital on a typical week day would be surprised how quiet it can get in the off-hours.

When the elevator doors opened, I pressed the button for the ground floor and quickly zoned out as the elevator began its downward journey. But when it touched down on the ground floor, the doors didn't open. Instead, the elevator went right back up again!

It stopped at the top floor. I waited a few seconds, expecting the doors to open. But they didn't, so I pressed the *open door* button and . . . nothing. I took a deep breath and got out my cell phone to call the postpartum front desk—there was always a staff member there—to ask them to send someone to help me.

But there was no reception. As a nurse, I'm used to keeping calm in hairy situations, but did I do that? Of course I didn't: I panicked. I had a sudden recollection of an episode of *The Fresh Prince of Bel-Air* when they were stuck in an elevator for *hours*. That was *not* going to be me!

I did what seemed like the next logical thing: banging loudly on the doors with my fists in the hope that someone would hear it echoing down the elevator shaft. When this yielded no results, I hit every floor button on the panel, like that famous scene from the movie *Elf*. The buttons lit up prettily like a Christmas tree, but still the elevator didn't move, and no one came on over the intercom. The elevator just hovered there stubbornly and silently. I tried not to think about the dark, multi-storey shaft below me.

Not wanting to create more of a fuss than was necessary, I'd been holding off hitting the red emergency button. But now a fuss was exactly what I wanted to make. When I pressed the button, it made a shrill, obnoxious ringing sound—a sound that apparently only I could hear. There was no phone in this elevator, so calling some mysterious control centre wasn't an option either. No one came. Nothing happened.

I did a few jumps, thinking how silly I must look on the video camera (there wasn't one), then crouched down against the wall—there's not a whole lot you can do in a small empty box—and stayed that way for what was probably five minutes, though it felt much, much longer. I started hearing funny noises, like an animal scratching, and the sound of wind—probably my mind playing tricks on me. I worked hard to ignore them as I sat down on the floor in defeat and put my head between my legs.

And then suddenly the elevator started moving. Hurray! But even though every button was illuminated, it headed down—to the seventh floor, where the doors finally opened. I was out of there like a shot, heading towards the stairs. There was no one around to hear my story, but at that point I didn't care. I just wanted to get home.

Since that day, the hospital has been renovated and the elevators replaced. But on the odd occasion when I go there, I still take the stairs. I can use the exercise—or so I tell myself!

ANOTHER INCIDENT OCCURRED at the same hospital when I was a nurse in the NICU. Babies whose health was deteriorating or who needed surgery often got transferred to the children's hospital across the street. To get there, we walked through an underground tunnel that, other than hospital and medical staff, very few people know exists.

The tunnel is long and straight and made of unfinished concrete, so it has that musty basement smell. The only illumination comes from industrial cage lights, which create eerie, intermittent pools of yellow with dark sections between them. There's no cell phone reception. I had heard stories about medical personnel who'd experienced a Code Blues or Code Pinks down there, which unnerved me. That worry, and the overall creepy atmosphere, can make the walk feel much longer than it really is.

The first time I used the tunnel, my mission was to transfer a newborn baby in an incubator. There was a ton of monitoring equipment, and a porter was sent to help me. I was relieved not to have to go through alone, although I didn't say so.

We were walking along silently, focused on our task and the baby in our care. The only thing we could hear, aside from the tunnel's ventilation fans, was the squeak of the incubator's wheels as the sound bounced off the cement walls. Around the tunnel's halfway point, an old-fashioned red phone was attached to the wall. A hotline to something, I supposed. No one had told me what it was for, or if I could use it.

We had just passed by the phone when it rang. The shrill, startling sound echoed through the tunnel. Should I answer it? Maybe it would stop. But no, it just kept ringing. Perhaps someone needs me, I thought.

Deciding it was best to err on the side of caution, I backtracked a few steps and picked it up. At first I heard nothing; then came the distinctive sound of heavy breathing. I hung up, spooked, and returned to the incubator, which I now pushed with a little more determination. The porter looked rather uneasy, but he didn't say anything, which made me wonder if this had happened before. It felt like I was crossing a rickety bridge that I was hoping wouldn't give out before I got to the other side. As we finally reached the end of the tunnel, the brighter lights, and the elevator doors with their cheerful SickKids logos, I breathed a huge sigh of relief. I had heard nurses say that the tunnel was creepy, but no one had mentioned anything like what just happened to me. (Nurses compartmentalize a lot of things, choosing not to share them. In my case, I didn't think anyone would believe me if I told this story.)

On the way back, I decided to cross the street above ground. There was lots of traffic, but on this occasion I didn't mind waiting for the light to change.

NURSE WITH GRIT

Mary Eliza Mahoney (1845–1926)

Born to freed slaves who came to Boston from North Carolina, Mary Eliza Mahoney became the first African American to earn a professional nursing licence. She graduated in 1879 from the New England Hospital for Women and Children, one of the first nursing schools in the United States, while in her mid-thirties. (Out of the forty-two women who entered the intense program, she was one of only four who completed it). Though she remained a lifelong advocate for Black nurses, rampant discrimination forced her to abandon public nursing for private practice tending to wealthy white families on the east coast. On August 18, 1920, the day the women's suffrage amendment to the US Constitution was ratified, Mahoney became one of the first women to register to vote in Boston. Although long retired by then, she proudly listed her occupation on her voter registration card as "Trained Nurse."

Amie

I've been present for hundreds of deliveries over the course of my career. I've even performed some myself. And if that experience has taught me anything, it's that there's no rhyme or reason for when births happen. I've delivered babies solo in the hospital when the doctor didn't make it in time. I've even helped women give birth in elevators and on sidewalks.

Thankfully, most of my experiences have been straightforward and unremarkable. But those aren't the stories people want to hear. Everyone always asks about the sensational ones. The screamers and drama queens. For me, the winner in that category, by a long shot, was Katie, a so-called birth tourist—meaning someone who leaves their home country to give birth in another—from overseas.

Katie arrived on the ward already shrieking, with a terrified look in her eye. But her scream wasn't that of a woman in labour; it was what you'd imagine someone would sound like if they were being stabbed with a butcher knife.

Though, like most nurses, I had training in what's called cultural competence, using it was a challenge with Katie, who didn't speak any English. There would be no "talking her down." (The birth was also imminent, so getting a translator was out of the question.) It's rare when more than two nurses are needed to deliver a baby, but to stop Katie from injuring herself we needed four: one to hold down each of her limbs, which were wildly flailing about. None of us had ever seen a woman behave like this. While flailing, she kept trying to shut her legs, which, needless to say, isn't conducive to having a baby.

Katie wasn't a small woman, and she kept managing to break away from our restraints. If her hands were free, she'd use them to yank out giant tufts of her hair. Or else she'd grab us, and her nails would dig down into our skin as we tried to break free from her grip. Several times she shook us off completely and starting crawling up the back of the bed. (I'm not sure where she thought she was going.) I kept thinking of Linda Blair in *The Exorcist*. It truly seemed like she was possessed! Her partner was also in the room, but he stood as far away as he possibly could, in the corner of the room. When we asked him to come over and help us, he was like . . . Nope, I'm good!

But babies, like water, always find a way. Despite her best efforts not to, Katie eventually did give birth. The amazing thing is that the second the ob-gyn put the baby on her chest, Katie fell dead silent. She went from completely unhinged to completely content, calm, and focused on her baby. She talked quietly and lovingly to her spouse, who had remained in the corner the whole time, witnessing her behaviour. It was as if someone had come into the room, picked up the remote, and switched off the blasting stereo.

WITH ANNA I got the opposite experience to Katie, volume- and demeanor-wise. Anna was my only silent birth.

Anna was tiny—five foot two at the most (her husband was tiny too)—so at nine months pregnant she was all belly. When she arrived on the ward in the early stages of labour, I was struck from the get-go by how quiet she was, especially since it was her first time giving birth. The only sound that came out of her was the odd, barely perceptible moan. In a pattern that was the exact opposite of virtually every other woman on this planet, she became quieter and quieter as the labour progressed, so much so that by the time I checked and found her fully dilated, she was making no sound at all. This silence stood in stark contrast to the (entirely normal) cacophony of screams happening all down the hallway.

When we spoke after she arrived, Anna talked about wanting to level herself by drawing on different energies. Her plan was to enjoy the birth process. She opted not to take any drugs or an epidural.

There's a fair bit of coaching involved with most women while they're giving birth. You have to remind them to breathe. Some will declare, "I can't do this," so your job is to convince them that they can. To be supportive and encourage them to draw on their inner reserves of power. To remind them how truly magnificent what they're doing is.

But Anna required no coaching at all. She kept her breathing quiet and controlled, essentially letting her body do all the work. I hadn't had kids myself yet, but I came out of that birth wondering if I could ever achieve a similar Zen-like level of control.

One of the most fascinating things about Anna's behaviour was the way it affected everyone else in the room. Taking our cue from her, we all fell silent as well, including her husband. On the rare occasions the two of them communicated, it was in whispers. For a while there I was convinced I could hear my own heartbeat. The whole experience somehow felt natural, despite the clinical atmosphere.

When the baby's hair was visible between Anna's legs, I called the doctor. When she walked in and saw, or rather *felt*, the environment in the room, she fell in line as well. The communal sense that we were respecting this person's unspoken wishes was palpable and powerful.

I assumed that Anna's demeanor would change during the pushing phase. I was wrong. Instead, the library-like quiet meant I could hear sounds I wasn't used to, like the clinking of medical instruments as the doctor did her prep. I could actually hear Anna's body doing its work, including the visceral whooshing sound the amniotic fluid made as she gave the last push. (Normally you see but don't *hear* the fluid.) The closest thing I can compare it to is isolated vocals after the instrumentation has been stripped out from a song. It had that kind of beauty to it too.

It was the cries of Anna's newborn baby that finally broke the hush. In the context of what we'd just experienced, the sound was overwhelming; it changed the energy in the room entirely. For the first time, Anna showed emotion, allowing tears of joy to fall as she held her baby in her arms. The baby's grandparents came into the room at that point and the entire family shared what I took to be some kind of traditional broth.

There's a saying in nursing: "Pain is what the patient says it is." With most patients, you see the pain in their face, the raw anguish. I don't think it was possible that Anna *wasn't* in pain, and yet the muscles of her face while she was experiencing it stayed relaxed. She closed her eyes but didn't scrunch them up or furrow her brow. I never saw her jaw clench, even during what's known as the "ring of fire"—that burning, stinging sensation when the woman is fully dilated and the baby's head is crowning against the opening of the vagina but she's not pushing yet. Arguably the most excruciating stage of birth, it's usually accompanied by a fair amount of vocalization from the mother.

Because they couldn't explain what they were seeing, several nurses thought there must be something wrong with Anna, or that she was on something. I felt instinctively that this wasn't the case, although I never did find out if she had planned her silent birth in advance. My experience with her was uncanny, almost magical. And like most truly special events, never to be replicated.

BECAUSE THERE IS a culture of superstition around labour and delivery, one thing we never do is jinx ourselves by talking about obstetrical emergencies during a shift. Another unspoken rule is that we never use the Q-word. If you arrive for your shift and see nothing on the nursing board, you *do not* say, "Ah great, it's gonna be quiet!" Saying this guarantees it won't be.

However, no one informed me of these rules when I was a novice nurse. I had to learn them the hard way. One of these learning experiences happened mid-shift on a very busy day. Since I was such a keener, I had printed off a bunch of documents about major obstetrical emergencies so I could study them. At some point, I turned to my preceptor, Danielle, with a question about cord prolapses (this is when the cord rather than the head is the presenting part during birth).

Danielle cautioned me about engaging in such talk on shift, but she went ahead and explained standard procedure in the case of a cord prolapse. She said the first thing to do was yell *"Cord!"* at which point nurses would come running like the cavalry. If you're attending the patient, your role is to stick your hands into the vagina—whether your gloves are on or not—and hold the baby's head off and away from the cord until you reach the OR. If you don't, the baby's oxygen and nutrients could get cut off, potentially leading to asphyxiation. Most women receive EFM (electronic fetal monitoring) during labour, a method that uses electronic instruments to continuously record contractions and the baby's heart rate as well as any fetal distress. Cord compression is something we see regularly in labour and delivery. There will suddenly be a steep decline in the heart rate, which we can see through EFM, whenever a body part—leg, bum, back, head, etc.—presses on the cord (if intermittent auscultation is used, we can also hear it). Heart rate declines are usually short and abrupt and no cause for concern. They become serious only if they happen frequently and for long periods of time, restricting the baby's blood flow and oxygen, thus risking fetal malnourishment, brain damage, and even death.

Some of the nurses who overheard this emergency talk were in the process of shooing Danielle and me away from the nursing station when we heard it. *"Cord!"* The coincidence being so unlikely, we assumed someone was pulling a prank. This assumption lasted about two seconds; by the third second, our asses were out of our chairs, and we were running towards the voice.

Tina, the woman in question, had come up from emerg in a wheel-chair and was in obstetrical triage, just a little way down the hall from labour and delivery proper. It was obvious she was in extreme distress, screaming and writhing in pain. She was heavyset, and we knew it would be a challenge to move her from the wheelchair to the bed. But we also knew time was of the essence.

We looked down between Tina's legs as she sat in the wheelchair in the triage bay. Instead of a cord what we all saw clearly was a foot . . . This baby was breech.

By now there were eight of us in the room. We'd managed to get Tina onto a bed and had called a Code Pink—the code for a baby that isn't breathing. We knew a Code Pink would draw the neonatal team (nurses and a pediatrician to help with any neonate complications).

The five beds in the triage bay were all occupied, each with a woman looking in horror upon the unfolding scene.

The biggest concern with a breech birth is that the baby might not be breathing when it comes out, so needless to say, tensions were high. Dr. Laurent, who was an OB, and the Code Pink neonatal team arrived, which was made up of three nurses, an emergency physician, and a pediatrician. With about fifteen people, the room was now packed and buzzing with anxious voices, the tension palpable.

Then Dr. Laurent cut through the din: *"Everybody shut the fuck up!"*

Dr. Laurent was new to the staff, and we didn't know her well. She had come from a New York City facility with what seemed like a superior, snooty attitude. While everyone else wore blue or green scrubs, she came to work dressed in tweed skirts and four-inch heels. She was unquestionably eccentric. The most generous thing anyone would ever say about her was that she was a "personality."

But now, here she was taking control of the situation and resetting the tone in the room in a way that took everybody aback. Even Tina stopped screaming.

"Hands off the breech!" Dr. Laurent commanded the now-silent room. "We're going to deliver this baby, but nobody is going to touch it."

I would learn only later that touching a breech baby's foot can cause the startle reflex, creating labour dystocia (the baby getting stuck). Delivering a stiff baby, let alone a breech one, is extremely challenging and requires a highly skilled obstetrician. Normally the patient would be taken to the OR so that an emergency C-section could be performed immediately if things went awry, but we were past the point where Tina could be moved.

Dr. Laurent turned to Tina and lowered her voice. "I'm going to stand here and watch this happen," she said.

The next one to two minutes felt like an eternity. Dr. Laurent got gowned up, but since it was too late to hook Tina up to an EFM, she performed intermittent auscultation, an alternative way of listening to the baby's heart via a handheld Doppler. She told Tina *not* to push—a massive challenge given how huge her contractions were.

The rest of us stood by feeling helpless as the baby slowly came out. And I mean *slowly*. We're talking ring of fire times ten. You could have cut the air with a knife. We looked on in amazement and admiration as Dr. Laurent managed to manipulate the baby's other foot out without touching the one that had already presented itself. The bum emerged shortly after, followed by the rest of the body, which was a terrifying shade of blue grey. The baby was whisked away by the Code Pink team.

Tina was taken to the ICU, where they checked her heart, which was showing signs of stress after the intense delivery, and repaired the brutal vagina-to-rectum tear.

But the next day mom and baby were both in the postpartum unit recovering. This was a huge relief. Tina's baby had been born so blue and limp that several of us had assumed it was dead. No one had ever seen anything like it.

Our respect for Dr. Laurent increased considerably after this (with the exception of a couple of nurses who had the nerve to complain because she swore during the birth). Most obstetricians aren't skilled in breech deliveries, but Dr. Laurent's expertise in the area was one of the reasons she was hired in the first place. In the same situation, a less-skilled OB (that is, most of them) would have gone straight for a C-section.

But as much as we respected her professional skill, Dr. Laurent was consistently abrupt to the point of rudeness. I don't think it mattered to her if she hurt people's feelings. I worked with her for a time at a colposcopy clinic (a colposcopy is a procedure to closely examine the cervix, vagina, and vulva for signs of cancer or other disease) where the clientele was primarily South Asian. There had been high rates of HPV in the community. When one woman asked how she could possibly have the sexually transmitted infection (many women in that community being virgins when they marry), Dr. Laurent didn't bother sugarcoating her response: "Ask your husband." The woman looked shocked.

Dr. Laurent often complained to the nursing staff about "shitty men" sowing their wild oats. She was a strong advocate of young boys and girls getting their HPV shots. Her opinions weren't wrong—but you might say her approach left something to be desired.

That said, I'll take Dr. Laurent—with her superior medical skills and sometimes abrupt bedside manner—any day over another doctor I worked with who became notorious for C-sectioning patients without giving them the chance of a natural birth. Worse, he was rushed and sloppy, and often left the surgical theatre looking like the set of a horror flick.

Physicians get paid a higher rate to perform C-sections than to perform vaginal births, as well as for deliveries that take place in the evening, so his motivation wasn't hard to understand. C-sections allowed him to control the timing of the births he oversaw and to keep that gruesome assembly line moving. The more the better, payday-wise. He would actually instruct us, "Keep the patient until 5 p.m., then I'll section her." Our complaints to management about this behaviour consistently went unheeded.

This doctor's C-section addiction led to some dicey situations, especially at night, when we typically worked with a skeleton crew that included a single anaesthesiologist. If we got two simultaneous emergencies requiring general anaesthetic, it would be up to the anaesthesiologist to make the call about which life to save.

My first C-section with him was memorable for all the wrong reasons. Although I'd already heard the horror stories about him from multiple nurses, I was still shocked and weak in the knees when I witnessed his uncontrollably shaking hand pick up a scalpel and plunge it into the woman's belly, causing blood to spurt out of her like a fountain.

More than once, he slashed a baby's head open with the scalpel so seriously that both baby and mother required stitches. (I remember the pediatrician who dealt with this case being furious.) Mind-bogglingly, he then expected his patients to show gratitude for his careless, endangering "work," and went as far as reprimanding them when they failed to thank him.

He treated nurses abysmally—that is, until he needed us on his side to cover for an error, or to appease our anger after saying something egregious or making us work three or four C-sections back-to-back. His go-to tactic was to buy pizza for everybody. I remember as many as ten boxes arriving on the ward at once, and he went out of his way to make sure everyone knew it was he who had bought them. But no one ever mistook these overcompensations for actual acts of generosity.

How did he get away with all this for so long? One major reason was probably familiarity. We tend to trust those who look like us, and he was a member of the Southeast Asian community, the hospital's largest client base. Many patients gravitated towards him simply because they thought he looked trustworthy, like their father or their uncle.

It would have been easy enough for him to attribute all the C-sections he performed to labour dystocia (slow labour), which is both common and hard to disprove after the fact, but sometimes he didn't even bother to pretend. A woman would be in the pushing phase, and he'd turn to a nurse and say, "I've got to leave now, so we're going to do a C-section."

The doctor's behaviour stressed everyone out. We all knew this wasn't how it was supposed to be. The complaints and outrage against him piled up, but for a long time no action was taken.

This finally changed in 2018, when he gave up his licence following an investigation by the profession's regulatory body into whether he had engaged "in professional misconduct and/or was incompetent in the practice of obstetrics and gynecology." Prior to this, he managed to get it back and, incredibly, he continued to practise. He was in his sixties by then and couldn't even get through an entire shift. He'd manage maybe six hours before asking another doctor to take over.

How was he able to profit off the pain of others for so long? It all comes back to hierarchy. He was respected but also feared, so the hospital kept deferring to him at a time when patient safety should have been their number-one concern. I saw the way nurses' complaints, including my own, were dismissed. Which brings me back to the importance of advocacy. Sometimes, speaking up for the vulnerable—like a woman delivering a child—requires butting heads with a few people. Like doctors. Doing this used to scare me. Nowadays it feels like an honour.

Nurse Q

*I*t's *July 2022, temperatures* everywhere are soaring, and Swardiq "Q" Mayanja, who prefers to be called "Q the Nurse," or simply "Q," is a bit bummed out. A few days ago, he explains in his distinctive Boston accent, someone broke into his grey Prius, the one that has taken him all over the US in the last two and a half years. It was the second break-in in three months. This time they stole his beloved roller skates and, oddly, a bottle of laundry detergent. Q arrived in San Francisco a month and a half ago for a three-month contract, his eighth assignment since he began travel nursing almost three years ago. He loves the Bay Area, despite the parking, which is hellish and expensive, and the city's very visible social problems—particularly homelessness, which is fuelling the kinds of petty crimes he just experienced. Q keeps his head shaved and his stubble groomed, all the better to highlight his bright, intelligent eyes. He loves skating in the various cities he visits. For the next little while though, he'll be walking.

Q is one of thousands of travel nurses in the US and Canada who regularly leave their home base—if they even have one—to take on short-term roles at hospitals, clinics, and other healthcare facilities. The requirements for travel nursing are pretty straightforward. Candidates are expected to have at least one year of experience in their specialty, which can be almost anything: med-surg, ICU, NICU, labour and delivery, telemetry. Q is trained in med-surg, but he has also worked in telemetry ("tele") and progressive nursing (also known as transitional care). Generally speaking, travel nurses are hired by specialized staffing agencies rather than directly by hospitals. Typical assignments run from one to four months, although at least one large academic health system, in Pittsburgh, launched its own in-house travel nurse agency during the pandemic. Its goal was to retain nurses while giving them the opportunity to work at other hospitals within their nationwide network.

Travel nursing is said to have originated in the late 1970s in New Orleans, when extra nurses were brought in from out of state to help care for the hordes of revellers who descended on the city for Mardi Gras. It's been on the rise ever since. Travel nurses cover maternity leaves, vacations, and sabbaticals, and deal with general staffing shortages. During the pandemic, when shortages were acute everywhere, the need for travel nurses exploded. In 2020 alone, the field grew 35 percent over the previous year.

According to workforce experts, there are enough licensed nurses in the US to fill all available full-time positions. But even before the pandemic, many were quitting due to dissatisfaction with their wages and working conditions. According to Bloomberg, before the pandemic, the University of New Mexico Sandoval Regional Medical Center had never used travel nurses. After the pandemic, the centre was paying $1.5 million a month for about sixty travel nurses at a time when the payroll for its full-time staff of 580 was about $3.3 million. Staff nurses have been increasingly quitting their jobs to take advantage of the flexibility and better pay offered by travel nursing. This has created a vicious cycle: when staff nurses quit, hospitals cope with the ensuing shortages by hiring—you've got it—more travel nurses. UNM Sandoval lost nearly a third of its 200 nurses to travelling positions during the pandemic, when its staffing needs were even greater. It coped by hiring travellers, some of whom were recruited from Canada.

A nursing assignment qualifies as "travel" if it's outside a 110 kilometre (50-mile) radius from a nurse's home. And while some nurses take on these shorter commutes, many go much farther, taking a plane, or like Q, their car, to faraway states and provinces. For a lot of travel nurses, distance is a major part of the appeal. Check out a travel nurse agency website and you might have a hard time telling it apart from a regular travel agency website. "Adventure Is Calling!" proclaims Travelnurse.ca, the website of Vancouver-based Solutions Staffing, one of Canada's bigger travel nurse agencies. On their splash page, there's an image of a woman—a nurse who's presumably finished her shift—sniffing the bouquet of a big glass of red wine next to the headline "Medical Professionals Wanted for Immediate Work." Other agencies prominently feature images of people mountain biking, scuba diving, and clinking champagne glasses against the backdrop of beautiful locales. There's a lot of emphasis on fun. On work, less so. Another agency suggests it can indirectly improve your love life. "Keep your mind and heart open," its website says, noting that travel nurses often meet their significant other while on assignment.

Q, who's in his late twenties, began his nursing career at a rehab facility in 2016. Although he was aware of travel nursing while in school, he didn't seriously consider it until a year into his job, when a colleague who had travel experience approached him and suggested he'd be good at it. She probably saw what we do: that Q has all the ideal qualities of a travel nurse. He's extroverted, with big energy and a natural ability to go with the flow. (It doesn't hurt that he's hilarious and good-looking too.)

When asked what qualities make a good travel nurse, Q says the most important thing is being willing to ask the "dumb" questions that others might shy away from. Simple stuff, like where to find supplies or how to log on to a hospital's computer system. Q's answer is kind of surprising. After all, if you're new, how can you be expected to know these kinds of things? Why would you be embarrassed to ask? "Nurses are Type A," Q says. "Sometimes you feel judged if you don't have your shit together. The majority are good, but if you meet the one nurse that makes you feel bad, it's demeaning."

Since travel nurses are always coming into a hospital that's in need or in crisis, they're expected to hit the ground running. There's no leisurely two- to three-week orientation, no hand-holding. The nurses you encounter, Q says, are likely to be stressed or at the burnout point. "Everything is tense, rough, shitty. That's the reason you're there. You've got to understand you're walking into a fire and you're there to quell the flames." When the situation is finally under control and the next group of nurses is hired, you're out.

Another big draw of travel nursing is the freedom and flexibility it offers. Unlike full-time staff in hospitals or other facilities, the travel nurse has a lot of control over when and where they work. Say they want to visit an old friend or attend a wedding or a music festival. They can try to tie an assignment to the city where those things are happening. And they'll travel there free, with the agency picking up the tab for transportation. It's a great way to knock a few things off their bucket list. But nurses also use travelling as an opportunity to expand their resumé and skill set in new environments or prestigious facilities. And they get more than a built-in vacation with their assignment; they can also take breaks between assignments.

Q loves the freedom and the adventure of travel nursing, but what he loves the most—"I'm not gonna lie," he says—is the money. Travel nurses can make a lot of dough, fast. Things were particularly insane during the pandemic. In January 2021, according to the American website ZipRecruiter, wages for travel nurses surged to almost three and a half times that of regular full-time nurses. Pre-pandemic, staff nurses at US hospitals made an average of US$1,400 a week. The typical travel nurse made US $4,000 a week. During Covid, however, some were making as much as $10,000 a week. Plug the hashtag #travelnurse into TikTok or Instagram and you'll see endless videos of travel nurses bragging about their newfound riches. One claims to have made $163,000 in thirty weeks. Others flaunt Louis Vuitton purses, Porsches, and the new luxury high-rise apartment they just moved into. All travel-nurse agencies offer to find their clients accommodations. These are usually very nice, but some nurses prefer to take the time to find cheaper digs and pocket the tax-free stipend. This is what Q does. And most of the time it's worked out well—with the exception of an assignment in Texas, where an apartment that looked nice in the online tour turned out to be a roach-infested dump. There were piles of dirt and dander from the previous occupants' animals. The neighbourhood was rough, with gunshots and drag racing a regular, distressing soundtrack. The couch was broken, its cushions ripped apart. Q cut his losses and got out as quickly as he could.

He loves doing corny, touristy things when he travels. He's learned more about the cities he's visited than he knows about Boston, where he lived for twenty years. In Texas, he attended his first rodeo, where he marvelled at the stagecoach races and the cattle with massive horns. For a city boy, it was mind-blowing. But he also loved the people, whom he describes as "amazing." Q is a social guy, so he'll go to parties and clubs, but he also loves early morning strolls and walking tours. In some cities, he's done two or three of these tours, just to get the full lay of the land. In Los Angeles he ran his first marathon. Several of the nurses on his contract were in a run club, and they encouraged him to sign up. (He jokes that he only agreed when he heard that the LA course was one of the flattest ones. He finished, but it was still brutal.) He's also done Spartan races, which are done in a field, with obstacles; and he recently completed a half-marathon that included an obstacle course. Wherever he goes, he stays active and engaged.

The assignments themselves have run the gamut. One of the best was his second, which was in a small community hospital in Maine. The work wasn't particularly exciting, but Q loved the nursing team. He subscribes to the adage "teamwork makes the dream work," and this team was as dreamy as they come. They showed him the sights and took him to restaurants. He formed a bond with the group and has managed to stay in touch.

Unfortunately, he's learned that not every assignment is that good. In some places the staff have been openly hostile. There can be a lot of drama. A contract he took in the Covid unit of a hospital in Greenwich, Connecticut, on the New York border, was, in his words, "toxic." It was the height of the pandemic, a time when all hands were needed on deck. Staff were terrified for their personal safety, but their boss was hiding behind a Zoom screen, trying to manage them from afar. Not cool.

Q HAS DEVELOPED a formula for approaching assignments. Once he's got the city pinned down, he makes a short list of possible places to live via a website specializing in short-term furnished accommodations.

Next, he fires up Facebook to find out who from his long list of friends lives there (this is when having a high school graduating class of 500 comes in handy). Next comes the ask, "Can you do me a solid and make sure this place isn't in the middle of a war zone?" After arriving in town, he returns the favour by taking the classmate out for lunch and, in the process, rekindling the friendship. It's a win-win.

Q was born in South Africa, but his parents are Ugandan, and he often draws on the resources offered by the large and far-flung Ugandan diaspora in which he grew up. Having six kids made vacations prohibitively expensive for his parents, so until he became a travel nurse most of Q's travelling was to the huge family reunions organized every summer, either in Atlanta or various Northeastern states: Maryland, New York, Massachusetts. Q uses the term "family" loosely. Of the two or three hundred people at a typical reunion, only about 10 percent would be actually related to him. The rest would be community members and close friends that he and his siblings and their many, many cousins referred to as "Aunt" or "Uncle." Q loved these gatherings, which involved renting out an entire floor plus the reception hall of a hotel. Food would be cooked and brought by local Ugandans: platters of fragrant brown rice, beans, and lots of chicken, beef, and fish stews. Q gets hungry thinking of it.

Q's mother is Christian, but he was raised in his father's religion, Islam (like many Ugandan marriages, theirs was arranged). In 2001, when Q was six years old, his parents, tired of South Africa's racist apartheid policies, moved to the US and settled in Newton, Massachusetts, just west of Boston (hence his accent). It was not what you'd call an ideal time to be a Muslim immigrant in America. But whereas in South Africa his family's Black identity had marginalized them, in the US, ironically, it proved an advantage—people saw Q and his family as Black, not Muslim.

In South Africa, Q attended a private Muslim school, or madrassah. Since this was not an option in Newton, Q went to the local public school, where he had no problem fitting in. In fact, he loved it. And the fact that he was Muslim rarely even came up. On the occasions when it did—if his friends came over and saw his family praying, or fasting for Ramadan—it never seemed to be a big deal. (It helped that Newton is a fairly liberal enclave.) "We had it so good," Q says dreamily. "In South Africa the racism was so blatant, raw, out there, that when I came to America and someone in a store looked at me or questioned me, I didn't even recognize it as bias. It was only later that people explained to me that this doesn't happen to everybody." He laughs. "When you're in Africa, the coolest human beings are Black Americans, so I thought I was on top of the totem pole. Not only did I feel that there were no racial situations, I also felt like I was the standard-bearer of coolness. So I'm grateful, I'm happy."

In high school, sciences came easily to Swardiq, and repeated aptitude tests kept giving him the same results: nurse, teacher, coach. Many of his relatives—aunts and uncles—were nurses, and his mom was a nursing assistant. The writing was on the wall: he'd follow in the family footsteps and become a nurse.

Like many nurses, Q initially got funnelled into medical-surgical (med-surg, as it's informally known). In any given hospital, med-surg is the most populated floor, this being where all manner of illnesses, whether chronic or acute, are treated. Q had been in med-surg for a year when his insightful colleague suggested he pursue travel nursing. At the time, Q was planning to move out of his parents' place, where he was still living. He thought about his friend's advice. "If I'm going to do it," he said to himself, "Why don't I do it big and actually explore life?"

He connected with an agency, which walked him through the process. It was more tedious than difficult. Different states required different licences, and each had its own rules and regulations. In California, for example, nurses can't have more than four patients.[1] They have to complete a new job application at minimum every three months.

Scrub colours and computer systems will vary, but the job of nursing does not: you treat a person who's had a heart attack in Massachusetts the same as you would in California. For Q, the only downside of being a travel nurse was being away from his family for so long. When we last talked, he hadn't seen them in almost three years. At that point, he had had eight contracts in four states—Connecticut, Maine, Texas, and California—with just one break after the hellish assignment in Connecticut. About half of his patients were originally from New York City. And while the city itself was an eerie ghost town, the second Q walked into the hospital he saw it was in complete chaos. As waves of patients with Covid symptoms flooded in, Q and the other staff were learning about the virus firsthand, on the floor. At the beginning, most of the patients coming in were in the forty to over-ninety age range. Then things shifted alarmingly. Young, otherwise healthy twenty-five-year-olds who had been playing basketball the day before were being admitted and immediately put on ventilators. When his first Covid patient was on his deathbed, Q had to lend him his cell phone so he could say goodbye to his family—all the hospital's devices were being used for the same purpose. It was the scariest experience of his life, and when he heard people questioning the seriousness of the virus it made him crazy.

Things came to a head when Q was told to use the same face mask for an entire week to compensate for PPE shortages. Until that day,

1   It would be safer for patients if these ratios were standard across all hospitals. Unfortunately, this is not the case. It's something we're fighting for in Canada as well.

the emphasis had been on maintaining impeccable cleanliness and throwing masks away after a single use. It now seemed as if his and his colleagues' safety wasn't a priority. So even though travel agencies were offering as much as $8,000 a week for contracts, he decided a breather was in order. He headed to Sacramento to lock down with a few friends who were sharing a house there. He stayed for three months, then found another travel gig just a couple of hours away in Oakland.

Q's parents are happy with his choice of profession, but the travel part of it not so much. They miss him when he's gone. When Q was growing up, like many immigrant parents they were on the stricter side. Q had a 7 p.m. curfew and was allowed to go to parties only on very rare occasions. It helped that during his teens he was a three-sport athlete who always held down a job in summer. "At the time I thought they hated me, but looking back I think they did an amazing job to keep us safe, to taste the culture without letting us go wild and loose. It was a good balance." The Western version of parenting, he says, is very different from that of many African and immigrant families. In North America, parents don't need to worry as much about their child's safety in a new culture, so there's more emphasis on being friends with their kids. Although that is slowly changing, he says. "In my family, my parents tell me what to do and I do it. This doesn't change just because I moved out or got a car. It's set in stone. But the older I get, the closer I feel to them as human beings."

One of Q's goals was to work in cardiac ICU. He found a hospital that was willing to train him over six months, with the expectation that he would stay and work for another six months. But this amounted to a full year and he wanted to keep travelling, so he turned it down. When we first spoke to Q in 2021, he'd been travel nursing for almost two years and wasn't sure if he could continue for much longer. The constant pulling up of roots was tiring, and he missed his family. His plan was to stop as soon as he reached his savings goal.

When we caught up to him a year later, however, he seemed to have a renewed sense of purpose and energy, his missing roller skates notwithstanding. Being single and in great health, he couldn't see a reason to give up travel nursing. He'd been on the west coast long enough that east coast weather was hard to contemplate. Would he settle there? Maybe—if he could convince one of his siblings to move out. The last time they had spoken, one of them sounded interested.

NURSE WITH GRIT

Agnes Chan (1904–1962)

Born Ah Fung Chan sometime around the turn of the last century (the exact date is unknown) in China, Chan was sold by her parents to a rich family as a young girl in the hopes that she would have a better life. She would be sold several more times, including to a family in Victoria, BC. But it was not a happy placement and, citing mistreatment, she eventually ran away to a Chinese missionary school. Now going by Agnes, Chan wanted to become a nurse, but there were no schools on the west coast willing to accept a Chinese student. Another missionary charity stepped in and arranged for Chan to travel to Toronto to attend the Women's College Hospital's School of Nursing, where she excelled in all her studies, particularly obstetrics. Her graduation, in 1923, made her the first Chinese-Canadian RN. Chan went on to do post-graduate pediatric nursing in Detroit, later returning to China, where, for a time during the Japanese occupation of the country, she ran a missionary hospital completely unaided.

Sara

The difference between nursing school and nursing in real life is the difference between theory and reality: school smarts and street smarts. You can only learn so much in a classroom. And a lot of what you do learn you never end up using in practice. I studied the principles of wound care, for example, but rarely applied them except during a brief stint in med-surg and while treating a patient with a rare infected C-section incision.

There were things I wish I'd been taught but wasn't. I learned lots about schizophrenia, for instance, but little about postpartum depression, which was far more common among the patients I spent most of my time with in labour and delivery. I would have loved to learn more about advocacy, a word that got dropped without any real concrete examples attached to it (except maybe Cathy Crowe). And no one ever told me about nurses' tendency to eat their young—that is, for experienced nurses to treat young newbies with hostility or even cruelty. It was only when I saw the opposite—an older nurse treating a newer nurse with warmth and hospitality—that I started to understand what was going on!

People often ask me if nursing school is difficult. My standard answer is: it's not difficult, it's *busy*. There are a lot of make-work projects whose sole purpose seems to be to cut into your scant personal time. For example, it was often suggested that we use our days off to research our patients ahead of clinicals, learn about their diagnoses, etc.—which I did diligently, even though it seemed a bit much.

When classes started, we hit the ground running and were immediately put into labs to practise doing intramuscular injections (IMs) on oranges. I can't say I was a natural at it, but then again, putting a needle in an orange is nothing like putting it in a human. Where human skin is elastic, an orange has very little give, so half the time the needle would poke right through the other side or come out bent. The best advice I got for giving IMs came later, from patients. One told me to throw the needle in like a dart (sounds scary, but it really works!). Others taught me to always inform them of what I was doing and not to take forever, the anticipation being worse than the needle itself.

Expectations of us were high, far higher than they'd been in high school. One thing I didn't anticipate was the thousands of pages of reading we were assigned each semester. I practically needed a wagon to get my textbooks home. The books themselves were also horribly expensive. It wasn't until third year that I realized I didn't need to buy the newest edition every time, that I could pick up older ones cheaply. I got smart about other things too. I initially spent hours doing both the required and the optional readings until I discovered that key points always got covered in class. The optional stuff I dropped in short order. If I was going to survive, I'd need to choose my battles.

Everyone seemed invested in their own success, whereas I, who at eighteen was still basically a kid, just felt stressed. I didn't feel comfortable participating in the library study groups the other students organized, or even engaging in post-test chatter ("What did you get for the question about the fourth cranial nerve?"). I remember doing a practice test and breaking down in tears because I couldn't remember any of the material.

But I was also too conscientious to fail. I started to settle down after the Christmas break in first year, and I even started enjoying my courses. We took many of the same basic courses as any doctor: anatomy, physiology, pharmacology. We learned about the body's workings, various diseases, and nursing interventions ("treatment" was a term reserved for physicians; nurses used "interventions" or "care plans"). We were taught how to determine when things weren't going well and when to get a doctor involved. My favourite subject was physiology. Our prof's analogy for how the kidney filters out toxins—dumping a bunch of spaghetti in a strainer—is still what I imagine whenever I get a patient with kidney issues.

We spent a lot of time on nursing theory. Too much, in my opinion. In the beginning I thought the subject might interest me, but a lot of it went over my head, and the rest seemed too abstract, not applicable to the real world. The theorists themselves struck me as boring, wishy-washy, and overwhelmingly white. (Nursing theory wasn't what you'd call a diverse field of study, something that doesn't seem to have changed much in the intervening years.) One of the most beloved, Jean Watson, had a "theory" of human caring that boiled down to the notion that it's good to be kind. Which is fine and true, but it also fed into the idea that nurses had to be angelic handmaidens and nurturers. Everybody except me seemed to love these theories though, so I rarely complained about them at the time. I didn't want to be the one raining on their parade.

In all four years we had 15 hours of class time and 15 hours of clinical practice weekly. My first clinical placements were at a hospital about a 40-minute drive from the university. Though it's relatively far south, this part of Ontario is also in the snow belt, so my main memory of these trips is of being squished in the back seat of someone's car going down the highway in nerve-wracking white-out conditions. (We were usually required to arrive on the unit by 7 a.m., if not earlier, to look through charts and get acquainted with the patients we'd be dealing with that day.) We carpooled to save money, and because many of us—including me—didn't have a vehicle. If you didn't have a car, or if your placement wasn't served by public transportation, too bad: the onus was on you to find a way there.

London is a major medical hub with several teaching hospitals, but I don't recall being given options for my placements. I was just told where to go. The situation seemed to be sink or swim, so I never questioned anything. I just kept my head down and put in my hours. Over four years I did placements in med-surg, long-term care, mental health, pediatrics (the latter at a daycare because the hospital's pediatric unit considered us too inexperienced to deal with the complex needs of its patients), oncology/hematology, and labour and delivery. At the end of each placement day we had a praxis, a sit-down with our clinical instructor to talk about what had happened. We were also expected to keep a weekly journal in which we reflected on what we were learning.

The advantages doctors are given over nurses begin in school. To become a doctor you need to do an undergraduate degree, followed by four years of medical school and a two- to five-year residency. You get paid during this residency. Nurses, conversely, are not paid for the three-month, full-time consolidation they're required to do in their final year of school, even though they work the same 12-hour shifts as preceptors, the experienced nurses who oversee their training. (Hospitals technically aren't supposed to use nurses-in-training as extra bodies.) This situation persists, despite a movement in recent years to eliminate unpaid internships in other fields, which are viewed as exploitative. Back then, we were often told we should feel grateful for these unpaid opportunities to work!

Clinicals is where the rubber truly meets the road, nursing-wise.

Initially, I mostly observed procedures and surgeries. In med-surg I watched a laparoscopic gall bladder removal and a coronary artery bypass graft (a common form of open-heart surgery).

I was also supposed to see an amputation, although this never ended up happening. The patient was a diabetic in med-surg who had gangrene in both feet. This being fairly rare, I was sent into his room at one point under the auspices of giving him medication so I could observe and learn. I know a lot of people would have been disgusted by the man's shiny, stiff flesh, which had turned a greenish purple from lack of blood supply, but I was fascinated. (I was okay with the visual, but not with the sharp, acidic odour rising from his feet, which was the reason he had a private room.)

When I observed the coronary artery bypass graft, they provided a stool in case I got lightheaded. But I didn't. As with the gangrene, I found the whole process completely fascinating. Before he was put under, the patient told me he wasn't nervous, that he trusted the doctor completely. I thought about those words as the surgeon broke the man's ribs with a shockingly loud *Snap!* using a special device. Think of the sound of knuckles cracking, but times a hundred.

Nothing we learned in class truly prepared me for the OR. This included how incredibly cold it was. My main reference point was *Grey's Anatomy* episodes. But on TV the camera angle is always at the head of the bed, through a viewing window on an upper level, which I have never seen in real life. Here, I was inside the actual theatre, about six feet from the patient's side. I was close enough to clearly see his cracked ribs and beating heart, the rest of his body having been draped off according to the principles of infection control.

I watched in amazement as scrub nurses placed instruments into the surgeon's open palm without a word being exchanged, as if it had all been choreographed in advance. (There's a strict pecking order in the OR, with the surgeon at the top deciding everything, from the exact placement and angle of instruments to whether to play music.) I was particularly struck by the contrast between the delicacy of the surgery and the seeming nonchalance of the staff. They chit-chatted about water-cooler stuff—gardening, cooking, their grandkids, none of which interested me in my early twenties. Still, hearing them talk this way relaxed me. I knew it meant everything was going as expected.

Another surprise was what anaesthetists did, or rather didn't do. Assuming everything went fine administering their meds, which were drawn up before surgery, their main role was to sit next to the patient's head and closely monitor them to ensure they didn't wake up. The job, like an airline pilot's, is 99 percent boredom and 1 percent sheer terror.

I felt at home in med-surg and could easily have ended up there. But after my final placement in labour and delivery I found myself fitting effortlessly into that world. This placement also made me realize that I preferred patients who were awake, not asleep!

WHAT I WAS learning in school often diverged from my on-the-ground experience. In class, teachers emphasized the importance of building relationships with patients, but in clinicals there was little to no time to do this. Once, on a rare occasion when I had a chance to do something not strictly required of me, I offered to wash a patient's hair (our textbooks said to always ensure our patients' hygiene was up to date). The patient seemed incredibly grateful and immediately said yes—it turned out no one had done this for her for weeks. It showed me that often it's the little things that help patients feel human in the hospital's sometimes dehumanizing atmosphere.

Some of the most difficult situations we faced were ones there was no training for. For example, during my consolidation I was sent in alone to provide care to a woman who had lost twins at 19 weeks. She was in deep grief, crying constantly. I had a lot of empathy for her, but that didn't mean I knew what to say or do, and this made me feel really uncomfortable. I was only twenty-one at the time, not yet a parent, and with no training in infant loss I was unsure if my presence was making things worse for the poor woman.

There was no nursing school class to teach me how to help the unhoused individuals I encountered, especially in labour and delivery. I felt terrible for these women who had no supports during such an important time in their lives. It was really them against the world. Many were racialized and felt judged by the healthcare system. Some had to take the bus to hospital while in labour because they couldn't afford a cab, let alone a car. They often arrived on the ward with a single bag containing all their earthly belongings. During the day, social workers were around to help handle these cases. At night, though, we were on our own.

I watched other nurses to see how they dealt with these patients. Some were matter-of-fact, others empathetic. But it shocked me how many were ready to judge and label them. The patients clearly sensed the nurses' disapproval. Some, especially those who had lost a baby before, had a strong distrust of the healthcare system and acted defensively. It was hard to blame them. One woman insisted that she didn't need any of the things we had to offer—extra help with breastfeeding, access to a social worker, diapers, wipes, blankets, even food from the cafeteria. She said she was used to being on her own. But childbirth is something no woman should have to face by herself.

It was when I started doing IVs that I finally felt like I was on my way to becoming a real nurse. Not all units give you the chance to build IV skills, so I was lucky to be placed in labour and delivery, where most women will need an IV. (The best IV nurses are found in emergency departments, where they poke people repeatedly.)

I learned to use different strategies for different types of veins—sick people's veins are never as good as healthy people's—and that there's a limit to how much poking a person will withstand. If you've tried twice with no success, it's time to get help from someone else.

There are few things as satisfying as hitting a vein in exactly the right place. There's a technique, even an art to it. In postpartum and in my job in clinical research, I drew lots of blood from adults. In the NICU I had to draw blood from babies, but never quite mastered it (unless you count heel pricks). Infants' veins are notoriously hard to find, so blood is usually taken via the hand, the scalp (which requires shaving the head), or even the foot (something that is never done to adults, as it can lead to clots). A crying baby is tense, so the first step is to calm them down, usually by getting them to feed. Next, you warm the chosen area and determine what size needle you're going to require. There's no chart for this. At one point the NICU acquired a vein scanner, which we were told was going to make our lives easier. But it was so inaccurate that it soon started gathering dust. Since you usually can't see the vein, you need to feel for it. This is where the art comes in.

I had a friend who wanted to be a nurse but who struggled to get through nursing school because she passed out when she saw blood. (There are many nursing jobs that don't involve dealing with needles and blood, but nursing school remains traditional in the sense that it requires exposure to blood and other bodily fluids.) Blood has never bothered me, but some smells really do. In the summer I often worked as a PSW in nursing homes, and as much as I liked the people, some of the odours really got to me, even made me gag. Once, somebody came into the hospital from a nursing home with a hip so badly broken that their entire leg was completely sideways. That I could handle. The smell of their diarrhea, not so much.

With mastery comes pleasure. I started to love drawing blood when I became confident that I could nail it every time. Which is not to say that it works in reverse. Paradoxically, perhaps, I *hate* the feeling of having my own blood drawn, no matter how skilled the nurse doing it is.

Inserting a catheter, like doing an IV, is another thing you can't really learn from a book. It requires practice on both men and women (women are harder). We were instructed how to deal with certain awkward situations, like when a man gets an erection (hand him a blanket and give him a minute). Fortunately, this didn't happen often in practice. Most women who get an epidural during childbirth require a catheter, so I became good at inserting them, but I can't say it's something I ever enjoyed.

I didn't realize while I was going through nursing school what a safe cocoon it provided, sheltering me from the realities of the profession. As a nursing student, you aren't the one ultimately responsible for your patients, since there is always a clinical instructor or a staff nurse to oversee your work. You don't have to make those tough beginning- and end-of-life decisions until you're in the thick of it. In nursing school, your biggest worry is whether you're going to pass or fail your clinicals or do well on your essays.

In real life, though, when you're a nurse people depend on your skills. Their lives are truly in your hands. There are those short-staffed days when you have to scramble to cope. Or you have a patient who objects to the plan of care you made for them. Or a family member who disagrees with absolutely everything you say. It takes time to adjust to the gap between a textbook's description of the way things are supposed to happen, and healthcare's messy, complex, frustrating, and sometimes inspiring reality.

Amie

I know I'm in the minority of nurses when I say this, but I *loved* working nights.

It comes down to the culture and the atmosphere. Night shifts are way less pressured and frenetic. During the day, hospital brass are never far away, and while I've been told night-shift managers exist, I've personally never met one. Magically gone too is the bureaucracy, the lining up along walls so politicians can do their photo-op tours, the huddles, the education modules, the diagnostics and imaging, and the million "important" things that keep you from getting your job done.

But here's the other thing: the (mostly) chiller night-shift vibe means we nurses get a chance to run the show and the autonomy to practise nursing the way we were trained. When emergencies happen, we pitch in and help one another. You'd think that day shifts would flow better, given the greater resources and staff at our disposal. But in my experience, it's the nights that unfold like a symphony—that is, a symphony whose conductor has temporarily left the podium.

Which isn't to say there isn't chaos. On nights in labour and delivery you still get Code Pinks and babies demanding to be born—especially if it's a full moon. I've never seen any official stats, but we all talk about it: when there's a full moon, wild and wacky things happen, and every woman seems to have her baby between 1 and 4 a.m.!

Occasionally, night shifts drag into day shifts. More than once, I've been with a woman who's pushing at 7 a.m. and the jerk nurse from the next shift refuses to come and take over, even though it's their job. If you add in the time it takes to catch up on charting after the baby is born, you might still be at work hours after your shift was scheduled to end. That said, there are also times when you want to stay with a patient you've bonded with, just to see things through.

And those bonds are easier to forge at night. My best, deepest conversations with patients have all happened in the wee hours. Maybe the mom-to-be is having her dinner and I'm just lingering in the room a little longer after an obstetrical assessment. It can be as simple as asking what your patient does for a living, sharing an anecdote or a joke.

That connection can include the patient's family, especially since the extension of visiting hours. When I started nursing, families had to be out by 9 p.m. at the latest. These days they can generally stay as long as they want, provided they're quiet and respectful of the privacy of other patients. Getting to know their family helps you see your patient in a different light. It can be a lovely, even profound experience for us nurses. And family members—whether a spouse, a parent, or a child—often jump at the chance to be involved in their loved one's care by helping to take them to the bathroom, for a walk, or to the cafeteria. Witnessing such intimate interactions has always felt like a privilege to me.

The best-kept secret, or maybe I should say the *worst*-kept secret, about night shifts is the naps. If you went to a day manager and said you were off for some shut-eye they'd either freak out or laugh in your face. During nights, however, napping is practised widely if unofficially on every ward—at least every ward I've ever worked on.

Let me be clear. We don't nap on night shifts because we're slackers. We nap because if we don't, our work suffers.

This is why we all work hard to protect those secret breaks. If you walk into a room during a shift and find a nurse asleep, you're immediately going to back out as silently as possible. Lots of newbie nurses come in thinking they're exceptional and that they'll just power through their shift. After working three or four night shifts in a row, though, most will start reconsidering that attitude. When 3 a.m. rolls around, your whole equilibrium starts to feel off.

Most nurses eventually master a skill familiar to Navy SEALs: the art of the power nap. It's something you have to teach yourself, but once you learn it, it never leaves you. I haven't worked a night shift in years, but to this day I can still nap on command. It's a real lifesaver if you have kids. Just a 15-minute micro-nap in the car (when I'm parked, or even while Jordan is driving me home) is all it takes to completely recharge my batteries.

And it's not like we're the only ones who nap. Physicians do it too. In fact, trying to find a doctor during a night shift can be a challenge, since they have a habit of not telling us where they're holed up! Doctors' sleeping spaces—so-called "call rooms"—are individual, fully equipped, and *way* nicer than ours, which often consist of a lounge with a chair or a loveseat (this is why we sometimes end up sleeping in patient rooms).

And even if you do know where a doctor is, you can't just barge in and wake them up. Summoning them requires a formal page through the hospital switchboard.

Some doctors simply say, "Don't call me on nights unless it's an emergency," which would be fine if their idea of an emergency were always the same as ours. Let's say it's 2 or 3 a.m. and your patient is in so much pain they can't sleep. If their chart doesn't have a standing order for pain medication, the only way to get it—even an over-the-counter drug like Tylenol—is to request it from the doctor on call. I can't tell you the number of times I and other nurses have been yelled at for what amounts to a policy problem. A labouring mother's pain might not seem like an emergency to a doctor in the midst of REM sleep, but I can tell you from personal and professional experience that it definitely feels like an emergency to her.

Doctors don't have to be in the building when they're on call. Most hospitals only require that they be able to get there within a half-hour. But there are always a few who go rogue. I called one doctor at night through the switchboard only to have his wife answer and put me on hold while they negotiated about whether he should come in. I've called others during the day who answered from golf courses that I'm pretty sure were more than a half-hour away. Then there's the ones who cavalierly say, "Just give them the drug and I'll sign for it in the morning." Um, no.

When it comes to sleep breaks, the difference between doctors and nurses is that doctors seem to have a sense of entitlement about them. I never felt I had the luxury, or the right, to say to a patient or a staff member: "Don't bother me, I'm sleeping!" I still had to check a woman who was dilated four centimetres every 15 minutes, regardless of how tired I was (this can go on for hours). But the toxic culture and the hierarchy in hospitals is such that often I was scared to call a physician in the middle of the night, even when an emergency was undeniable. For example, if you get an abnormal fetal heart tracing and are truly concerned for the baby's wellbeing, a doctor is required to come in to do an assessment. There are guidelines and standards of care that we're *all* supposed to follow, not just nurses.

In another typical scenario, the doctor comes in to check the patient, then announces they're going to a call room to sleep. Fifteen minutes later, the patient is feeling butt pains. When we check, we find that labour is progressing so quickly we have to call the doctor back. The doctor is annoyed—as if we nurses could decide when the baby was coming!

The mistreatment, the condescension, the ostracism—sometimes it just didn't seem worth it and we'd end up hedging our bets. But the situation was almost always lose-lose. No matter how much we complained about disrespect, there were never any consequences and the doctors' behaviour didn't change. We were often left feeling like punching bags.

The more experienced I became, the more intentionally I communicated my concerns to doctors. They hated it when I said that I had looked at a dodgy tracing and decided it was fine, that they needn't bother to come and assess the patient. Labour and delivery is a highly litigious area of practice, and I've seen MDs deflect the blame for disasters by claiming that the nurse never told them how bad the situation was.

I think my interest in advocacy began when I was working night shifts. The calmer space gave us all a chance to express grievances and strategize about issues. Night shifts also gave us time to share and process the inevitable bad experiences and the traumas that are part of the job of nursing. You're supposed to debrief when something horrible happens on shift—like a maternal or neonatal death—but on night shifts this rarely happened. It was almost like we had been forgotten by our leadership team.

On rare occasions, I'd come in for a night shift and there'd be zero patients. When this happened, the nursing leader usually asked if anyone wanted to go home. But most of us opted to stay, knowing it would be one of the easiest shifts we'd ever work! Patient-free night shifts could also be pretty fun.

Some nurses used the time to shop on their phone or catch up on the news. Others took their "break" early and slept the whole night. Still others just chatted: about politics, healthcare, family. For years, there was a running joke about how lazy night-shift nurses sat around playing cards, ignoring their patients' calls for help. Let me be clear: I've *never* seen nurses play cards! And we weren't slackers. Anything task-oriented—restocking rooms, making checklists for OR supplies, or checking the Pyxis for medications—always got done.

After which there were the shenanigans. We'd get up to some crazy-ass stuff on those quieter nights. A particularly memorable one happened during Christmas week. Since many of us were working over the holidays and couldn't celebrate with our families, a few nurses had brought their unopened presents in. One got a hoverboard—those self-powered things you ride while balanced on a terrifyingly small platform between two wheels. None of us had ever ridden one or knew how they worked. This didn't mean we weren't willing to learn!

Six of us took turns riding, or attempting to ride, the thing down the long hallway next to the nursing station. Most attempts ended in crashes, some of them pretty spectacular (the only patient was on the other side of the ward and wouldn't have been able to hear us), with nurses landing bruisingly hard on their bums. We tried to record it all, although holding our phones was difficult given how hard we were laughing. Needless to say, if management had suddenly decided to walk in, we would've all been fired on the spot. They tried to get me to try it. I wasn't scared of getting busted, but there was no way I was risking my life on that thing!

Wheelchair races, on the other hand, I was totally up for. When it comes to having fun, a wheelchair is a hot commodity, and that night we had three. An entire fleet! The first type of race was the simplest:

whoever got to the end of the hallway first was the winner. The others were more like what you'd call chariots of rage, a kind of wheelchair roller derby in which you tried to bump the others off the "track" or throw them off their groove.

(NB: This was a *rare* occasion. Nurses are in general very responsible people, but sometimes even we need to let loose a little. There were no patients around when this happened, and no wheelchairs were damaged during the races—though there were definitely some squished fingers. Those things are built like tanks! Further, the wheelchairs were for use only in labour and delivery, so no one who needed one would ever have gone without.)

Another great part of night shifts was feasting. With one team in particular, I'd arrive for work and the first question would be, "What are we ordering tonight?" The delicacies would start to arrive between 1 and 2 a.m.: hot wings, samosas, slushies. This was on top of the ridiculous amount of food staff brought in, all of which reflected our eclectic backgrounds: Indian, West Indian, Portuguese, Italian, Serbian, Polish—we were a United Nations of nursing potlucks. I have such fond memories of that team.

There's a strong sense of comradeship in nursing, a bit like what you find in the military. You need to be accepted by the pack before you can begin trying to change things. At the time of the hoverboard incident I was a green bedside nurse, and I still felt the need to gain the trust of my colleagues, who had been together for a while and were tight. I wasn't going to break my neck on that infernal device, but a potluck dish I could do! (White-bean chili, anyone?)

On day shifts you're not supposed to bring in food because of infection control rules. The rules probably applied to night shifts too but we never bothered to check, and honestly we couldn't have cared less! Eating together wasn't just fun; it also increased our sense of camaraderie, which in turn revealed the strength of the team as a whole. I've always thrived on that sense of unity and shared purpose.

That good feeling often got paid forward. Part of the job when working a night shift is to restock supplies and set things up for the day shift, when resources get depleted much more quickly. We would do this, but then take it further by completing tasks that weren't strictly required, like checking temperature probes, or making sure oxygen settings were correct for babies that might need neonatal resuscitation during the day. We made cute hats out of the standard hospital ones or put together little care package for families. We made the rooms look like hotel rooms by providing "turn-down" service. One nurse knew how to fold towels into swans. I'm sure the day staff assumed this was done by the cleaners, and that was fine by us. We didn't do it because we wanted thanks, but because we knew how many interruptions the day shift faced, how little time they had to do any of it themselves.

If I ever went back to the bedside, I would choose to work only nights again for one main reason: if you want a truly collegial team, that's where you'll find it.

NURSE *WITH* GRIT

Loretta C. Ford (b. 1920)

After serving as a nurse during World War II, Loretta C. Ford went to work in the community. In this role, she became aware of the healthcare deficits and physician shortages in many communities, particularly rural ones. She and her nurse colleagues initially tried to address these deficits by setting up temporary clinics in schools and churches. But Ford was convinced that more could be done to make healthcare more accessible to the public. In 1965, she joined forces with pediatrician Henry Silver to co-found the first pediatric nurse-practitioner model and training program at the University of Colorado. The profession, which empowers nurses to develop medical plans for patients independent of doctors, has since expanded to all corners of healthcare in the US. (Sadly, NPs are severely underutilized in Canada, where millions of people lack a primary-care provider.) Ford also developed the unification model of nursing, which seeks to provide nurses with a holistic education through a combination of clinical practice, education, and research. At age 102, Ford is still an active member of the American Association of Nurse Practitioners, serving as a consultant and delivering inspiring lectures.

Nikki Skillen

*R*N *Nikki Skillen has* an emergency brain, which is why fifteen of her twenty-five years in nursing have been spent in emerg. Nikki calls herself a reactor by nature: someone who brings a thick skin to work and thrives when things get raw. "I function best in shit is the way to put it," she says. Nikki, who is in her early fifties, has a deep voice, wavy blond hair, and a demeanor that exudes calm confidence. She's seen a few things, and she's got the war stories to show for it.

One of the most memorable incidents in a career full of memorable incidents happened when she was working in triage—always the first point of contact for a patient coming into emergency—at a large hospital outside Toronto. The emergency room alone was 80,000 square feet, bigger than a football field. It was around 2 a.m. and the shift had been a typical one, as far as any night shift in emerg can be called typical. Nikki had just finished triaging an elderly woman with chest pain and was preparing to take the temperature of a feverish two-year-old sitting on her mom's lap. She looked outside and saw a man who appeared to be in his early twenties running up the ramp towards the hospital wearing just a pair of pyjama pants. He was screaming and swearing his head off. "Here we go," Nikki said under her breath.

With a decade of nursing under her belt, Nikki had developed certain instincts. In triage, for example, she could look at a person having a bad episode and immediately assess what type of drug they were on. Estimating that the ranting man would be through the hospital's three sets of glass doors in about two seconds, she ushered the mom and her little girl through a small door that would put them safely inside the registration booth, basically a big square box with a window.

The man was now inside emerg, his screams ricocheting off the walls of the unit. Nikki could see that beneath his dishevelment he was good looking and well cared for. He demanded to go to Four Main, the hospital's mental health ward. Nikki told him this would happen, but he needed to see a doctor first.

The young man seemed not to register this. He was now telling Nikki he needed to go to the bathroom, so she summoned security from across the hall to escort him there.

Nikki resumed triaging. A senior couple had arrived. The wife explained that her husband was having chest pains. Nikki listened to her, but out of the corner of her eye she sensed motion: someone was running towards her, and she didn't need to look to see who it was. She told the man with the chest pains to move aside, to the outrage of his wife, who seemed to think his condition wasn't being taken seriously. A second later she turned and saw what Nikki was seeing, and she and her husband managed to get out of the way before they could be accosted by the disturbed young man, who was now back in front of Nikki.

She needed to get him off the unit, but before she could do anything, he lifted up his arm and launched something at her through the sliding window that separated him from the triage area. She ducked, but too late. The object, which was spongy and wet, grazed her cheek. Nikki turned to look behind her and saw something on the floor that looked distinctly like a bloody penis.

Her emerg brain kicking in, Nikki strode out of the booth, grabbed the man by both arms, and dragged him through the doorway beyond the triage area that led to the examination rooms. She spotted the physician on duty, who was busy charting. "I need you in OR 4 right now!" she commanded (OR 4 was the hospital's biggest trauma room). When the physician didn't immediately react, Nikki clarified the situation: "Dude just cut off his penis."

Now fully aware of the situation, the physician moved to take one of the man's arms from Nikki and to remove his blood-soaked pyjama bottoms. The man resisted, but the doctor was having none of it. "Fuck you, those pants are coming off!" He grabbed both sides of the pyjamas, yanking them down while simultaneously tackling the man onto a stretcher. Meanwhile, Nikki attempted to slow the man's bleeding by manoeuvring one hundred pounds of sandbags onto his groin while another nurse used her own weight to simultaneously apply further pressure and get an IV in him. A few minutes later, the man went into cardiac arrest. Another nurse was called for.

Nikki was bent over the man, trying to hold him still, when the thought hit her. "Did anybody grab the penis?" she yelled.

The silence that followed was her answer: it must still be lying on the floor back in triage. When backup arrived, Nikki ran over to get the penis. A severed digit would normally be put on ice, but she was concerned the member might get frostbite (this is years before Prince Harry talked about his frostbitten "todger" in his memoir), so she decided to wrap it in gauze instead.

Nikki and her colleagues took turns using their weight, combined with the one hundred pounds of sandbags, to stanch the man's bleeding until he could be transferred to a hospital that specialized in the kind of microsurgery he was going to need. After the transfer, Nikki worked the rest of her shift, unaware of the blood smear on her cheek. Later, she would find out that it had taken four hours for the man's penis to be successfully reattached.

The full story would become a subject of conversation among hospital staff for the next month: the young man had entered the bathroom and severed his penis with a razor blade, leaving the bathroom looking like a murder scene. Given the man's obviously compromised mental state, security should never have left him alone.

Most of us will hear a shocking story like this and laugh nervously. (Emerg nurses will be the first to tell you that indulging in dark humour is essential for keeping their sanity.) But at its core is the very serious issue of how the healthcare system handles people with mental health problems.

DURING HER HEYDAY in emerg, Nikki was a nighthawk. This was by choice. As a single mother of two young children, working nights was easier because she could leave her kids overnight with her parents. After doing this for fourteen years straight, however, she developed severe insomnia and decided to make the move to ICU, where the shifts were more flexible, the patients less demanding and unpredictable, and where she finally felt able to fully utilize the nursing skills she'd spent years acquiring.

Even though you're dealing with critical patients in ICU, it's nothing like emerg. The environment is much slower and more controlled. There's no chaos; one patient alone will run you off your feet. An ICU nurse can be assigned a maximum of one vented patient or two non-vented ones (although sometimes a chronic vented patient will be paired with a non-vented one).

For Nikki, the adjustment was a challenge at first. ICU and emerg nurses think in totally different ways. In emerg, you have to react immediately to anything and everything that comes through the double doors. Unless the patient has something obvious, like a broken leg, your job is to figure out why they're there. Is it their chest? Their heart? Their breathing? And the conveyor belt never stops. As soon as one patient is stabilized, you're on to the next.

In contrast, ICU patients are assessed from head to toe. Any little thing has the potential to affect survival: that bruise on your patient's arm, the red mark on their butt.

ICU is the domain of nurses: doctors don't go into the patients' rooms to make assessments; they base their decisions on the assessments the nurses give them. (Nikki is just fine with this.)

The hospital where Nikki works, known by staff as "the mothership," is a Level 3 ICU with thirty-two beds. (A Level 2 facility won't take patients requiring ventilatory support; these get transferred to Nikki's hospital.) Ninety percent of ICU patients are unconscious and on life support when they arrive on the unit. Some are in medically induced comas or under heavy sedation because they're restless, fighting, coughing, or shivering, all of which drain precious energy needed to stay alive. Contamination is a major concern with these patients, so Nikki monitors hers from a distance, through a window looking into their room. Since there's rarely anyone to cover for her, it's not unusual for her to be at a patient's bedside for 12 hours straight with no bathroom break. To support organ function, patients are usually hooked up to machines such as ventilators, dialysers, and heart pumps. Because all this machinery creates pressure that forces respiratory droplets into the air, Nikki does what's called "clustering of care," meaning that she performs as many interventions, procedures, and administering of meds as she can at once in order to reduce her exposure. (She got really good at this during Covid.)

ICU patients are often unable to talk, so Nikki spends a lot of time communicating with their families. At some point, she'll need to broach the delicate topic of resuscitation, especially if no DNR (do not resuscitate) order is in place. She'll ask the family if they think their loved one would want measures like chest compressions, blood trans-fusions, defibrillation, or vents, or if they'd prefer a natural death. (If no orders are in place, the default is for all resuscitation measures to be taken.) It's not an easy conversation to have at the best of times, let alone when people are facing one of the most devastating, stressful times in their lives.

Medical science has progressed to the point where people can now be kept "alive" for an almost indeterminate period. And more life-prolonging drugs are being developed all the time.

But just because we *can* keep terminally ill people alive doesn't mean we should. Nikki gives the example of patients who come to her riddled with cancer. Many don't have the blood pressure needed to handle inter-ventions, which means the drugs they'll receive in ICU may actually kill them, or simply prolong their suffering. She understands that families sometimes aren't ready to say goodbye, so she sees part of her job as get-ting them to a place of understanding where they're ready to do just that.

She mentions a recent study on obtaining DNRs that followed two groups of doctors at a chain of hospitals. One group used a script when approaching patients and their families about a DNR; the other group didn't. The script itself used very specific language that made reference to allowing the individual to have a natural death, to decide what their body could and couldn't tolerate. Physicians who relied on a script got 90 percent more DNRs than the ones who didn't.

But sometimes all the listening and explaining in the world won't make a difference. Some family members insist on every possible intervention regardless of how severe or terminal their loved one's condition is. Which is why Nikki and her colleagues will sometimes end up breaking the ribs of a ninety-year-old while performing CPR on them.

The case of sixty-seven-year-old Hardeep sums up some of the troubling ethical questions that have become part of Nikki's daily reality. Hardeep had come to Canada from India to visit his pregnant daughter in the lead-up to the birth of his grandchild. He was making himself useful, working on the roof of his daughter's house, when he fell off a ladder and broke his neck. The accident rendered him an instant quadriplegic.

Hardeep was on a ventilator when he came to Nikki's ICU from another hospital, where his neck had been fused and stabilized. He later ended up with a tracheostomy. It took a while to wean him off the vent, but he eventually managed to go a month with no supplemental oxygen. Nikki was preparing Hardeep for a transfer to the wards when he started having problems with secretions in his lungs. Patients in this position simply don't have the energy reserves required to expel stuff from their airways on their own, and it was clear Hardeep was going to need an artificial cough assist.

Hardeep spoke English well enough to make it known that he was okay with ventilation for resuscitation, but that he did not want life-saving drugs or CPR were his heart to stop. There were multiple notes on his chart confirming this.

A few nights after he was put on the cough assist, Hardeep's heart rate started dropping. When Nikki came on shift, she found his daughter at his bedside, so she went to her with the intention of offering sympathy and to confirm Hardeep's DNR. The daughter immediately started screaming at Nikki while pointing to the DNR: "I never signed this!" She demanded to see her father's doctor. He confirmed that an intervention could not be performed without Hardeep's permission, but he assured her that her father would of course be supported if he were in any kind of distress. This discussion took place in front of Hardeep as he lay in bed, barely breathing.

Hardeep's daughter was furious. She started yelling that she had power of attorney, that she would sue the hospital. A POA is indeed able to override their loved one's wishes, so in the end the hospital was obliged to perform more interventions on the dying man. The fact that people don't always have final say in decisions about their own body is something that bothers Nikki a lot.

The question of money and healthcare can be awkward, but it has an ethical dimension too. Just lying in an ICU bed for a day costs more than $3,000, or approximately three times the cost of the average inpatient hospital stay (and it is ever increasing). Everything else— nurses, respiratory therapists, social workers, dietitians, specialized ICU meds to maintain a normal heart rate and blood pressure—costs an additional $20,000 to $30,000 a day. Hardeep had no travel medical insurance, so the financial burden of his care was borne by the Canadian taxpayer. Medevacking him back to India would have cost $50,000, a comparative bargain. (According to Nikki, if the same thing had happened in the US under similar circumstances, Hardeep would have been back in India inside of a week.)

Hardeep was kept alive, but it wasn't pretty. He ended up with necrotizing fasciitis and a bedsore so massive that most of his buttocks had to be cut off. The only mercy, Nikki knew, was that he felt no pain (this isn't always the case). Hardeep would lie in that bed until he finally expired and that, Nikki knew, could take a while.

People like Hardeep's daughter might change their tune if they could actually see what lies ahead for their family member. Keeping a person artificially alive slows down the dying process, but it doesn't stop it altogether. Some of Nikki's patients are on vasopressors, a class of powerful drugs administered only in ICU that divert blood from the extremities to the core to maintain organ function. Nikki likens the process to squeezing out a big wet towel.

The problem is that the extremities end up starved of blood, which leads to nasty stuff like toes and fingers turning black and falling off. Ten days in, a patient's arms, legs, and feet will start to go necrotic. Then come the venous stasis ulcers (open wounds) on the legs and, perhaps most horrific of all, tunnelling wounds: wounds that literally "tunnel" from the surface of the skin through the muscle or subcutaneous tissue. These can be surprisingly long, deep, and multi-branching.

Nikki had only been working in ICU for about a month when she pulled down the blanket of a patient on vasopressors and saw several of his toes fall onto the bed. The patient was a man in his mid-70s whose family wanted the hospital to take every measure possible to prolong his life. Nikki questions if you can call it a life. After a couple of months, the smell of this patient would hit her the minute she walked onto the unit. There was no candy-coating the fact that his body was rotting.

Sometimes patients are in the ICU because they need the temporary help of a ventilator to get over a critical illness (Covid being a prime example). If a patient doesn't show signs of turning around after a week or so, however, their chances of survival decrease drastically. Even the muscles of someone as young as forty will start wasting after three or four days of being bedridden. The longer a body is kept alive via machines and drugs, the more it becomes dependent on them. Other patients will go back and forth between ICU and the wards for months.

These days, most of Nikki's work is in a form of critical care called Rapid Response. Every Level 3 ICU in Canada and the US has a Rapid Response team consisting of a nurse, an internist (physician), and a respiratory therapist who will respond to any nurse's or physician's request for an ICU assessment.

Rapid Response is a pretty exclusive club. Like a secret society, you can't decide to join, you have to be invited. Part of Nikki's role in Rapid Response is to help families fully understand their loved one's prognosis so they can make informed choices about what comes next. For patients with little to no chance of recovery, that often involves explaining why a DNR may be the most humane choice. Because Nikki takes plenty of time with patients and their families, listens to them carefully, and uses sensitive, appropriate language to explain their options, she's often more successful at this than the physicians she works with. Strange as it may sound, this is the part of her job she enjoys the most and takes the most pride in. "We have to give them the info to make an educated decision," she says. "When you're pushing this on someone and the physicians want to do it quickly and get on to the next one, they're not putting any compassion behind it. They'll say, do you have questions? But families hear this as, do you want us to kill your family members or save them?"

One of the reasons Nikki likes Rapid Response is that it gives her back a bit of the reactivity of emergency, which she still misses. She loves the challenge of getting a new patient, a person who is deteriorating, and assessing how quickly she can turn the situation around with her knowledge, skills, and judgment. And unlike most nurses, she has the experience and the tools at her disposal to do so. As a member of Rapid Response, she can order her own X-rays, IVs, fluids, EKGs, and bloodwork, and use the results to perform her own interventions without consulting a physician (she particularly loves reading X-rays). Being able to work so independently helps make up for the fact that she's bound to a pager, and that there are still days when she won't get a bathroom break.

Another way Nikki and her team head off ICU admissions is by performing critical care interventions at the bedside to prevent crises like cardiac arrest. If, on the other hand, the patient is at the point of no return and essentially staring down death, she'll secure them a quick admission to the ICU.

She'll also do the opposite: follow patients discharged from ICU into the wards to make sure nothing goes wrong. (For example, a diabetic who has become acidotic [DKA] and is on the verge of a coma needs to go to ICU for 24 to 48 hours to stabilize before they can be sent to the wards.)

Nurses who have been in the job a long time sometimes experience burnout. Not Nikki. Her job in ICU allows her to use the full complement of skills she's acquired over decades, and she loves it. She feels confident and rarely second-guesses herself. She's also as tough as they come—an ICU and emerg boss *has* to be. But don't mistake this toughness for indifference. For Nikki, a good day can mean seeing a patient who came in unconscious with a traumatic injury get discharged with a second chance at life. But it can also be helping a family understand why they need to let their loved one go. Sometimes providing care means looking people in the eye with kindness and saying difficult things they might not want to hear, lending the ear that doesn't have the stethoscope in it.

Amie

In the house where I grew up in Brampton, unexplained phenomena used to happen all the time. Just ask my cousin Matt, who experienced them firsthand and is convinced to this day that the place was haunted. (Matt is also a nurse, and he shares a pretty intense ghost story of his own later in the book.) There were constant creepy sounds, a TV that turned on when no one was in the room, and dogs that barked mysteriously at the basement door (the tenant had recently moved out and they died a few weeks later). It got so bad that at one point my mom got a friend to "cleanse" our basement (this seemed to consist mainly of throwing salt around). I was raised on West Indian folklore about ghosts and evil apparitions; these were known as "duppy stories." And although I became more skeptical about these things as I got older, my cultural upbringing and my later experiences as a nurse made it hard to shake my belief in the uncanny.

When my grandfather was in palliative care, the other three men in his room died before he did. One day when we went to visit, Grandad was in an unusually bad mood. When we asked what was wrong, he said, "That asshole next to me won't stop bugging me." But the asshole in question (who wasn't *really* an asshole—he had a brain tumour that made him behave oddly) had died five days ago. Another man in grandad's room kept seeing dead relatives before he died himself.

Did I want creepy, inexplicable things to happen to me? I did not! The best place to experience the supernatural, IMO, is from the safety of your couch, or a theatre chair, bag of popcorn at the ready.

The first time I experienced something inexplicable at work was during my very first placement as staff nurse in labour and delivery. It was the night shift, and it wasn't busy, so we were all sitting around the nursing station.

People associate initiations and hazings with frat houses and the military, but new nurses get "initiated" too (usually, but not always, less violently). I'd been on the job for less than a month, so the timing was right. The nurses, who weren't the usual team I worked with and came across as a kind of "mean-girl crew," were telling labour and delivery stories that had taken a tragic turn. Seeing that I wasn't really paying attention to my book but was getting pulled into the stories, they called me over. One of them turned to me with a serious look. "Hey, Amie, you should know that we've had three maternal morbidities here." She went on to tell me that all three had occurred in Room 144. Convinced that the room had some kind of curse, the nurses now used it only for C-section prep, not deliveries.

Despite being green, I knew that maternal deaths were rare. But here were my colleagues claiming they'd had three maternal deaths in rapid succession in a single year. One was caused by a congenital issue the patient was unaware of. With the two others, the reason was an amniotic embolism, a rare condition where a woman's water breaks internally, allowing amniotic fluid to enter the bloodstream. When an amniotic embolism occurs, there's not much you can do; even with all the medicine in the world on hand, the patient usually dies.

My colleagues told me that the last woman to die in Room 144, which was along a corridor that led to the unit's operating rooms, had already delivered her child. New moms are checked every 15 minutes before being transferred to postpartum care. In this case, during the first check the mom already had her baby on the breast and seemed to be doing fine.

But when they entered the room for the next check 15 minutes later, they found the woman dead. Attempts to resuscitate her failed. Chillingly, her baby was still attempting to nurse at her breast.

The woman died, but she never left. That night my colleagues told me that multiple nurses had seen or heard her roaming the halls, looking for her baby. Labouring patients hadn't been put in Room 144 since the incident.

Though I doubted their story, I have to confess it made me uneasy. I'd never liked using that corridor. The lights didn't work properly, and the atmosphere as a whole was just whack.

It was 3 a.m. when the nurses finished telling me this tragic, creepy story. I and some of my colleagues had been scheduled for a rare three-hour sleep break. But when I looked at the list to see what rooms were free for my nap, only one was available. You guessed it: Room 144.

Although my heart was in my mouth as I wrote my initials next to the room, there was no way I was going to show any fear. I figured it was exactly what they wanted out of this newbie.

I gathered up my blanket and pillow and headed down the long hallway. My feet felt like lead. Room 144 was the last room before the ORs, which are kept extremely cold compared to regular ward rooms. This proximity—or so I reasoned—meant Room 144 would be freezing too.

I pushed open the door, which was big and heavy for infection and noise control, and walked into the room.

In front of me was the expected sight: a bed with a curtain around it that was pulled back. Beside the bed was a couch for visitors and a window that looked out onto a parking lot. I closed the door, but before getting into bed, I hesitated. Should I draw the curtain? Indecisive, I drew it halfway. Feeling paranoid, I also turned on the bathroom light. It didn't help that the room was freezing, even with a warm blanket on top of the regular bedding. I was so cold that, in my mind's eye, I could see my own breath. It felt like a room in winter. I needed to block it out, close my eyes . . .

Miraculously, I fell asleep. Then, maybe 15 minutes later, something woke me up. There was a big red clock on the wall, but without my glasses I'm as blind as a bat. As I felt around for my glasses, I had the sudden, strong impression that something was in the room. "Omg," I thought, "it's actually happening to me!"

I panicked. The room was darker than it should have been, and I realized why: the bathroom light had been switched off. But what made my heart stop was this: the curtain had been fully pulled around my bed.

I heard breathing, then realized it was my own. I was psyching myself out! I felt a kind of sleep paralysis, like something was on top of me, about to smother me.

I jumped out of bed, ripped open the curtain, and ran into the hallway. No one. I went back into the room and turned on all the lights. There were my glasses on the night table. I put them on and finally saw the time: 3:33 a.m.

My colleagues were surprised (or were they?) when they saw me back at the nursing station before my break was over. "Were you afraid you'd miss your shift? I would have come to get you!" one of them claimed. They said I should go back and catch a bit more shut-eye.

"That's okay, I'm *good*," I said. I'm sure they could detect a bit of an edge to my voice, but I didn't tell them what had happened.

My story, when I eventually told it, would join the legend of the unit over the three years I spent there. It got passed along by many others. So much so that even when I returned after an absence of four years, it got told back to me!

Sara

I spent most of my nursing career in postpartum. Known informally as the mother-baby unit, it's where we help mothers who have just given birth to prepare for their discharge home. You meet all kinds of people in labour and delivery and postpartum. There's no real "type," unless you count humanity itself!

Sometimes it's the personalities that stand out in your memory. Like the new mom who demanded that her baby be bathed at a certain time of day (why?), or the one who "ordered" tea with a slice of lemon from me. Yet another complained that the hospital breakfast was too high in sugar. For all these women I had a straightforward answer: "I'm here to care for you, but I am not your maid!"

That said, if a mom with a baby in the NICU asked me for a cup of water with ice, or if I could watch the baby while she went to eat, I would generally do it. Having an infant in intensive care is stressful. A lot of parents in this situation get a hotel room close to the hospital, but if a room happens to come available on the ward, we will offer it to them.

Our job as nurses is to care for all patients, regardless of their beliefs and presenting situations. We cannot refuse care to a patient just because they make choices we don't agree with—referred to in the profession as moral distress—or that we think may not be the best course of treatment. Some of the most challenging situations for nurses involve patient autonomy and ethical choice, both of which are important and integral to healthcare. It can get messy.

I have dealt with these situations while treating birth tourists (women who leave their home country to give birth in another). Most women come here not because our healthcare system is so great, but because they want their child to have Canadian citizenship. (Citizenship isn't a birthright in all Western countries. In the UK, for example, citizenship by birth is only automatic if one of the parents is already a UK citizen.) These mothers usually come here for several weeks, maybe rent a condo downtown, and head straight back home as soon as possible after the birth. The births themselves aren't covered by universal health insurance, of course. Most parents happily pay out of pocket. The hospital bill is cheaper in the long run and it's a surer way to secure citizenship than going through immigration routes.

(To be clear, birth tourists are not refugees. Refugees are usually fleeing their country of origin to escape war or persecution, and their healthcare would be covered by universal health insurance.)

Birth tourists are easy to spot. And some have shockingly privileged attitudes, possibly because they come from areas of the world that offer a combination of private and public healthcare. One woman came while in labour and demanded a private room on the grounds that her husband was a physician in their home country. She was screaming as if she were in mortal pain, but when we checked her she was only one centimetre dilated!

Some patients or their partners, convinced we had hidden private rooms, tried to slip us cash to secure one. (Women in active labour get their own room; what these birth tourists wanted was a private post-partum room.) Bribery being commonplace in many countries, they often seemed surprised when we told them not only that we couldn't take their money, but that there really were no hidden rooms.

When someone asks for a private room, our standard response is that we will add them to the list, but there are no guarantees one will become available. (In Ontario, OHIP entitles you to a ward room with four beds. When I worked in labour and delivery, private and even semi-private rooms cost around $350 or $450 per night.) One husband, a physician, was outraged by this answer and demanded to talk to the manager. When the manager confirmed what we'd said, he stormed off down the hall, opening doors. He was obviously hunting for empty rooms, convinced we were lying. He came back to say he had found one, but his smugness reverted to anger when we told him the room was already booked. We had no idea how to handle this kind of belligerence. Should we call security? Talk him down?

The cultural barriers we experience with birth tourists can be a bit head-spinning. One example was Nasrin and her husband, who had travelled from overseas to have their baby. Nasrin did not work outside of the home. Her role was to have children and maintain the family and house. Her husband earned the money, made the decisions, and was in control of all situations for the family. Nasrin and her husband seemed to have very defined gender roles in their marriage.

Every time I asked Nasrin if she had any questions, or if she needed help with the baby, her husband would jump in and answer for her. It got very weird. In a rare moment when we were alone, I asked her if she wanted privacy from her visitors so she could breastfeed the baby. "Ask my husband," she said. Questions about her level of pain were the only ones she would respond to directly. But when it came to medication to cope with the pain, she again deferred to her husband! I consider myself an open-minded person, but I found their dynamic very hard to understand. In my experience, many men don't know what to do with themselves while their partner is giving birth, or when it comes to anything related to breastfeeding, so I wasn't surprised when Nasrin's husband decided to stay out of the room during that period. To be honest, I was relieved.

Birth tourism used to be rare, but it became so frequent at one hospital where I worked—which was no coincidence, as it was conveniently close to the airport—that we had a series of staff meetings to figure out how to handle it. One thing we did was work with the communications department to make it clear on the hospital website that anyone coming to Ontario to give birth without health coverage needed to arrange payment with the finance department in advance.

Perhaps unsurprisingly, many people ignored this message. Non-citizens continued to show up at the hospital in labour and we scrambled to accommodate them. Some falsely claimed they had insurance. Others clearly took advantage of the system, knowing that we would never refuse them care. Time and again, birth tourists were allowed to walk out the door regardless of whether their account was paid. Call it a birth-and-dash.

Regardless of the reasons behind the practice, when a birth tourist skips the bill, it's the Canadian taxpayer who foots it. And the figures add up. In Canada, the cost of a vaginal delivery can be as high as $25,000, depending on the level of care required, even higher if the baby needs to be admitted to NICU. (In the US, the privatized system is set up for this. Bills are itemized and include all supplies used during a stay; everything has a bar code.)

Hospitals tend to service the ethnic and cultural communities where they're located, and these groups often have their own unique ways of responding to the birthing process. One suburban hospital where I worked had a large South Asian population, a culture where the mother-in-law has a lot of sway over the treatment of the newborn, whether it be feeding or holding it (the mother-in-law usually holds the baby). Mothers-in-law often came in to bottle-feed and bond with their grandchild, and allow mom some needed sleep.

The downside is that mothers sometimes opted not to breastfeed if their mother-in-law was against it. This shocked me at first. After all, breastfeeding is the healthiest option for a baby. However, in many parts of world, breastfeeding isn't a health issue, it's a class issue. Some see it as a practice that only poor people follow. Bottle-feeding is thus a status symbol, something only people with money can afford.

Wanting to change these misconceptions, we printed flyers in various South Asian languages extolling the benefits of breastfeeding and placed them in hallways, ward rooms, and bathrooms. I was not at that hospital long enough to find out if the messaging worked. But consistent messaging is always the first step in increasing breastfeeding rates.

At the other end of the spectrum from birth tourists are the patients who fly in from smaller areas, including Indigenous communities in the far north that don't have access to the kind of specialized care available in urban centres.

Annie was an Inuit woman from a town of 400 people in Nunavut called Sanirajak. There was concern that her baby might have a kidney condition requiring intensive care, observation, and antibiotics. Annie and her husband came to Toronto when she was 35 weeks pregnant and were staying at a nearby hotel while they awaited the birth. They had never been to the city before and seemed overwhelmed. To make matters worse, they didn't know anyone, and there were communication barriers. They struck me as isolated and a bit depressed.

Eating was a problem. The food available nearby was not suitable for them, and the hospital couldn't accommodate their diet. I was surprised at how informally they were treated; there seemed to be no care plan for them. It seemed like they didn't know what to do or whom to ask questions. So I took it upon myself to give them lots of information, as did the social worker, who put in extra time and effort to give them as much support as she possibly could. The information went both ways. The visitors were proud of their traditional practices, and I was interested, so I took the opportunity to learn as much about their culture as I could.

Happily, their baby was born perfectly healthy. We had some wonderful moments of connection, like when I observed them cuddling with the baby and offered to take their picture. They were given the green light to go home soon after. Not knowing what was available in their community, I packed up a ton of supplies: bags of diapers, wipes, formula, nipples, bottles, sanitary pads. I hoped they wouldn't see this as charity and be offended. But I needn't have worried. They were incredibly happy for all the care they received.

PEOPLE OFTEN ASK me what is the largest number of children that I've known a woman to have. That's an easy question to answer: thirteen, and none of them were twins. The mother, Rachel, was a patient in her mid-thirties. In labour and delivery, the term for a woman who has had more than five children is a grand multipara. Giving birth more than five times puts a woman at risk for a number of conditions including postpartum hemorrhage, so it's definitely information healthcare providers need to be aware of.

Rachel was a lovely person and an exemplary patient. She knew what she wanted but was never demanding. During the birth, she was amazingly calm and matter of fact, despite opting not to have an epidural. She seemed to take everything in stride. She didn't eat hospital food the entire time she was with us; every day, the religious organization she belonged to delivered to her room meals that looked and smelled delicious. Whatever she didn't eat she put in the fridge for later.

Rachel and her life fascinated me. There were a ton of questions I wanted to ask, and I snuck them in here and there in the conversation so as not to appear to be prying. One of them was: Where are all your kids while you're in hospital? She told me the boys had been placed with one family, the girls with another.

I was also curious how she managed at home with them all. She told me there was a certain efficiency of scale, with older ones helping younger ones, and other community mothers were a strong source of support. Like most women in her religious group, she wore a wig that she never took off in front of others, including me. Instead of a hospital gown, she wore an elegant traditional dress. Her husband often dropped by, but never with any of their kids. I didn't get a chance to ask what kind of work he did, but I wondered that too.

Rachel told me none of her children had required training to breastfeed. Her technique was to take each one to bed with her for three days after they were born and let the breastfeeding happen spontaneously. To ensure they got their fill, she "topped them up" with bottled formula after the breastfeeding session.

She said this so confidently that I didn't dare say what I was thinking, which was what I had been taught: if you're breastfeeding you should *only* breastfeed and never use a bottle. Doing both at once can cause nipple confusion and, worse, compromise mom's milk supply. The richness of formula in combination with mother's milk can also stretch a baby's stomach out. I knew all this, but I kept my mouth shut. Rachel's confidence and experience reassured me that she knew what she was doing!

She seemed very happy in the hospital, so happy that on the day she was discharged she asked if she could spend a couple of hours longer with us before calling for her ride. And who could blame her? Compared to a house with thirteen kids running around, this must have felt like a quiet oasis.

Before my patients go home, I usually joke with them, "So hey, maybe I'll see you in a few years?" With the birthing experience still fresh on their minds, most women will answer with an emphatic *no*. But when I made this joke with Rachel and her husband, they looked at me sincerely and replied, "Yes! Hopefully we'll be back. We'd love to have more children!"

Another patient who really stayed with me, albeit in a less good way, was Cindy, a woman who had had triplets via C-section. Cindy was an older mother, I'd guess in her early forties, who had conceived via IVF. What was unusual about her birth was that all three babies were a good healthy size, which meant they could be moved to the postpartum floor. Most multiples end up in the NICU, usually because they're born prematurely or are experiencing respiratory distress or hypoglycemia (low blood sugar).

Any one of Cindy's triplets could have been a single birth. That should have been a cause for celebration, but even though everything was fine with her babies, Cindy was incredibly rude and demanding. She ordered her husband and me around as if we were her servants. It was as if, in her mind, her job was done and now it was everyone else's turn to step up.

There were three little cots in the room so the babies could sleep next to her. But when they cried, she refused to get out of bed to pick them up or change their diapers. Instead, she'd call me to come and do it. If a mom is incapacitated in some way, then I'm always happy to help. This was not the case with Cindy, so I would tell her I was busy with other patients and simply couldn't provide the level of support she was asking for.

Her queenly attitude extended to feeding as well. I encouraged her to breastfeed and even brought in a lactation consultant, but she stubbornly refused to try it. At one point, clearly annoyed at my badgering, she said, "Sara, these are my babies, and I'm going to do what I want with them."

I asked if she was planning to bottle-feed them. "I'll decide later," she told me testily. All she wanted to do was sleep. Later, she told me that she'd decided to bottle-feed, and yet she continued to lie there flat on her back. "If that's the case, then can you sit up and do it?" I asked. The sense of combativeness I got from Cindy was continual and exhausting. The irony is that if the babies had been in the NICU, where there's a lot more staff, things would have gone much more smoothly.

In fairness, it can be hard to get up after a C-section. But Cindy didn't seem to want to. She didn't seem all that interested in the children themselves except when it came to their breathing, which she kept asking me to check. I'd oblige her, and each time they sounded fine. One did end up having respiratory problems a day or two later, however, and had to go to the NICU. This fuelled Cindy's anxiety even more, and she became super anxious about the other two.

Surprisingly, there are no written rules about whose job it is to bottle-feed babies in the hospital. That's because it's usually not an issue: most parents *want* to feed the newborns and be involved in their care. I would show a parent how to feed their baby once or twice, and they'd take over as soon as they were confident enough. The transition was usually quick and conflict-free.

Not with Cindy. When it came to feeding the triplets, her first choice was always for a nurse to do it. Her second choice was her husband, who came across as quietly compliant. (He actually seemed a little scared of her.) Their dynamic was interesting, to say the least.

When her husband went home at night, she'd start putting pressure on us again. Maybe she was planning to step up once she got home, but I have no idea if that's the case, since she told me more than once to butt out of her feeding plans!

ONE OF THE toughest things we deal with in both labour and delivery and postpartum is cases of intimate partner abuse and child apprehension. It's unusual for a woman not to want her partner present at their child's birth or to have a restraining order against them. If there is a restraining order, we usually get an electronic note telling us not to disclose the patient's real name to anyone who came by or called. On paper, charts, or binders, we used a pseudonym. Hospitals are less secure than you might think. Police and security guards aren't present on every floor. And when I worked in postpartum, a lot of the security systems in place were less than perfect. For example, all babies were supposed to be fitted with a security bracelet to stop them from being stolen from the unit (it happens), but the bracelets were always slipping off the infants' feet, or were so sensitive that they'd set off the alarm when the baby was brought too close to the exit.

Patients sometimes arrive on the labour and delivery ward with a Children's Aid Society alert. The most common reasons are addictions or substance-abuse issues, transience or lack of housing, or a history of intimate partner violence (IPV) or child abuse. Because the hope is always that the child's apprehension will be a temporary arrangement until the family can get the help they need, the CAS will try to place the child with a family member like a grandmother or an aunt. When this isn't possible, the baby is sent to a foster family.

Jane was a patient in this situation. As a courtesy, it had been arranged for the baby's father, whom Jane was no longer with, to have a single visit with the child before she was taken into CAS custody. But we also had credible information that the father might try to abduct the child, so we were all on high alert. The atmosphere on the ward was really tense. Security guards were stationed at both of the hospital's entrances, something I had never seen before.

I was keeping busy charting, checking on my other patients, and giving medications when the father arrived. He was tall and skinny, with dark hair pulled into a ponytail, and he wore a leather biker jacket. He appeared to be extremely on edge and kept pacing the halls. The baby was in her car seat, ready to go, Jane having already said goodbye a bit earlier. It was a sad scene. As the dad finally approached his daughter, we sat there holding our collective breath, trying to prepare ourselves for any scenario. When the father mumbled a few words to her and then left, we breathed a huge sigh of relief.

These are challenging situations for all of those involved, and nurses don't typically know the full story. Many of these decisions are made long before the patients arrive at the hospital. We simply try to support the patient and the family—say, by scheduling a meeting with a social worker—as best as we can.

Many cases that involve abuse are less clear cut. I suspected, but couldn't be sure, that my patient Gabrielle, who had just given birth to her second child, was being abused by her partner. I knew he verbally abused her because it happened in front of me and the other staff. The two of them would begin snapping at each other the minute he walked into the ward. He was aggressive and physically intimidating. If Gabrielle asked him to do something for her, he refused. It could be something as small as passing her the baby's diaper. He'd tell her not to be so lazy, to do it herself. He constantly called her stupid. He'd bring their other child with him, a two- or three-year-old girl who was often completely out of control, yelling, crying, having peeing accidents. This, more than anything, tipped me off that something bad must be going on at home.

It's a nurse's responsibility to intervene when abuse is suspected, but doing so is never easy. Patients are often scared or defensive. But I knew I had to do this with Gabrielle. So one morning before her partner arrived, I got up the courage and approached her. I tried to be discreet, but it was awkward to say the least, especially since she was in a shared room and the other women could hear everything we said.

(Later, it occurred to me that I could have written her a note. Of course, in a perfect world, every patient would have a private room—confidentiality is incredibly important to us nurses—but in most hospitals, especially on the postpartum unit, this isn't the case. Sometimes we get lucky and find a quiet meeting room where we can have a private discussion, but most of the time we improvise. Finding creative solutions for challenging situations is something a lot of us pride ourselves on.)

Gabrielle didn't answer me, but her eyes told me all I needed to know to take the next step and bring in a social worker. The social worker agreed that there was almost certainly something going on, but unless abuse could be proven, all she could do was give Gabrielle some resources and hope she followed up on them. We both knew the chances weren't good. IPV is complex, and sadly, many women never manage to break the cycle of abuse.

A situation like Gabrielle's is another example of the moral distress nurses face on a regular basis. Standards of care specify that the nurse-patient relationship must end when care does, which means that we rarely get closure in situations where we are concerned about a patient's wellbeing.

Due to their legal duty to care, nurses cannot refuse patient assignments. But it doesn't always work the other way around. Patients can and do refuse to have certain nurses assigned to care for them.

I've only been fired by a patient once. Nina was a woman with a petite frame and a short blond bob. She arrived on the postpartum floor in extreme pain after a routine C-section. Nina had no underlying health issues and her baby was fine, so we brought in a pain specialist and an anaesthesiologist to look at her. They came up with a detailed care plan, but nothing in it helped. The pain remained a constant and a mystery.

Women are often encouraged by their midwife or doula to make a birth plan. Reasonable as this sounds, in my experience women who arrive on the maternity ward waving a birth plan may as well be waving a red flag: they are almost always high maintenance. Maybe it's the pressure of too-high expectations, but these women always seem to have the worst deliveries, whether it's a C-section or something about the baby that lands them in the nursery. Nina had a birth plan, but nothing was going according to it.

It's impossible to know what someone else is feeling—in healthcare we always say pain is what the patient says it is—but it seemed to me that Nina's postpartum experience wasn't all that different from other women's. The difference was in the way she was—or wasn't—handling it. Like a lot of new moms, she experienced pain when she began to breastfeed, but instead of working through it, she declared right away that she was going to bottle-feed (I always ask parents what their plan for feeding is and support their wishes, whether it be breastfeeding, bottle-feeding, or both. At the end of the day, the most important thing is that the baby be fed!) Nina was definitely a type-A personality: direct and difficult to please. She was extremely irritable and bossed her husband around constantly. He did what she asked, but it never seemed good enough.

The only people she didn't treat badly were the doctors. To them, she was invariably polite and friendly, so much so that she almost seemed like a different person.

She saved her anger and frustration for the one who administered, rather than prescribed, her meds: namely me. She treated me as if I were completely incompetent and a source of her pain. I had spent days running back and forth getting her various medications—by now she'd transitioned from pills to injections—when she turned to me, her eyes fierce, and said, "I can't look at you anymore. You need to go."

I went to the charge nurse and told her that I'd been "let go," that she needed to assign someone else to Nina. I admit I felt a little rejected. I had never been fired from *any* job before. But the feeling didn't last. It was clear that Nina's issues were about her, not about me.

I warned the next nurse about Nina. She lasted until the end of her shift. I found out later that Nina came back to the unit to have her second baby. I can't say I was sorry to have missed it.

NURSE *WITH* GRIT

Dr. Leigh Chapman (b. 1973)

Nurses lost an important seat at the federal table when the Canadian government eliminated the position of Chief Nursing Officer in 2012, following years of underfunding. So it was thrilling when a decade later they not only brought the position back, they chose Dr. Leigh Chapman to fill it. Despite a career spanning twenty years in multiple nursing environments, Chapman was never an obvious choice. When someone floated the idea that she could become CNO, she told them she didn't think she would pass basic screening for the position! Like Cathy Crowe, Chapman spent years working on the nursing front lines with people society tends to cast aside: those suffering from poverty and addiction. She not only vocally criticized the government's response to the opioid crisis, she also personally established an unsanctioned safe consumption site in Toronto. When she was appointed, Chapman declared that her top priorities were improved working conditions and retention for nurses, as well as making them more active participants in discussions of health policy. And as the badass gritty outsider she is, we have no doubt she's going to do exactly that.

Cathy Crowe

*I*t's December 2000 *in* the east end of Toronto, and a middle-aged woman in a silver puffer coat stands on a post-apocalyptic-looking patch of land strewn with garbage and covered in sparse vegetation. Strands of blond hair from her pixie cut poke out beneath a red headband. Her face is obscured by a scarf and sunglasses, and a megaphone she's holding up. As she speaks, vapour rises from her mouth, a testament to the frigid weather. Standing around her are people far less warmly dressed. Some hold mugs with warming drinks. A fire burns in an empty oil barrel, fuelled by what looks like construction debris.

A massive flatbed crane truck becomes visible in the background and slowly starts beeping its way towards the group. Nearby, a few police officers brace themselves to stop it. They're unaware that, thanks to the lobbying efforts of the woman in the puffer coat and city councillor Jack Layton, the owner of the property where they're standing, American big-box company Home Depot, has just given permission for the truck to unload its cargo. This consists of prefabricated homes for some of the fifty people who have been living on the site in refugee-camp-like conditions.

"All systems go!" the woman yells through the megaphone. "The houses are coming into Tent City!" One of the units is slowly lowered to the ground, revealing a banner with the words "Disaster Housing" on its side. The woman declares victory to those gathered here, although she's under no illusion that this is anything close to a final victory. A longer, harder road lies ahead.

WHEN THEY MADE Cathy Crowe, they threw away the mould. This is one badass nurse you don't want to be on the wrong side of! Cathy is often referred to as "the original street nurse," a nickname that was, fittingly, coined by a homeless man. He meant it as a compliment, and that's how Cathy took it. In fact, she embraced it for the inherently political statement it made. The very fact that a specialty like hers existed in the first place was proof of how bad things had gotten.

When people think of "nursing," they're likely to think of a figure—okay, a woman—at a bedside in scrubs or a white dress and cap, depending on the era. Maybe she's setting up an IV line or taking a pulse. People are unlikely to think of someone like Cathy, who fights for her clients' rights to housing and food, both of which were listed as prerequisites for health per the landmark 1986 Ottawa Charter for Health Promotion. Sometimes she's even the one providing them.

Bedside nurses will often advocate for patients who can't speak for themselves because they're ill or unconscious, or because their family doesn't grasp the severity of their medical situation.

Cathy Crowe's patients are silenced because many live on the margins of society or are unhoused. They are people who often don't have a family member to stand up for them. People who, because they don't have an address, don't have a medicine cabinet, can't get "home" care, and often receive discriminatory care in hospitals or doctors' offices.

For the tireless work she's done for over thirty years with this population, Cathy has received a boatload of awards and honorary doctorates. She's also one of only a handful of nurses invested into the Order of Canada.

She's run for elected office twice, and although she lost on both occasions, the thing about Cathy is that even when she loses, she wins. When she ran for the Ontario New Democratic Party in a 2010 by-election, for instance, she leveraged her candidacy to save 119 precious palliative beds at a Salvation Army hospital in Toronto that were slated to close due to government mismanagement.

Cathy doesn't think of social justice and advocacy as add-ons to her job, something to do in her spare time. She thinks of them as intrinsic to her vocation. This attitude, and her copious achievements, has landed her in many Canadian nursing school textbooks. She has changed people's ideas about what a nurse can be, including ours. These days, we're honoured to be able to call her a friend and an ally.

NONE OF THIS happened overnight. Cathy, now in her 70s, has worn many nursing caps over the decades. She's been a cardiology nurse, camp nurse, office nurse, clinic nurse, community health nurse, nurse practitioner, primary care nurse, public health nurse, outreach nurse, and street nurse. But these job titles tell very little about her accomplishments, a list of which would fill a book. Actually, they *have* filled a couple of books, including her excellent memoir, *A Knapsack Full of Dreams* (2019), which should be required reading for all nurses, and anyone really. (The title is a reference to one of Cathy's heroes, Tommy Douglas, the father of Canadian healthcare, who was once described as having a "suitcase full of dreams.")

The knapsack in question was a black one that Cathy carried when she worked on the streets and did nursing outreach clinics in shelters and drop-ins. It typically weighed thirty pounds, loaded with the supplies you'd expect a nurse to have—stethoscope, thermometer, bandages, medications—but also many you wouldn't. Items like granola bars and Ensure for the malnourished. Tampons, socks, and transit tokens, which most people on the street don't have access to. People were so fascinated by her knapsack's contents that in 2000, Cathy started bringing it along to the many presentations and speeches she was being asked to give. It has since become part of a permanent nursing exhibition at the Canadian Museum of History in Gatineau. You can view it and its contents online.

Becoming a street nurse and an activist was a necessity rather than a choice. Cathy grew up in the Ontario communities of Cobourg and Kingston, in a happy, comfortable middle-class home that recalls the show *Leave It to Beaver*. Her mother, Jean, was an emergency room nurse. Her father, Bill, was a salesman for Mr. Christie's cookies. Cathy was only five when she decided she would follow her mother's vocation.

Although theirs was not what you'd call a political household, fairness was an important family value. Cathy's grandfather, Alex MacInnis, was a railway worker who fought for justice and equality as a member of the socialist Co-operative Commonwealth Federation (CCF). And Jean was often disturbed by things she observed at work, such as understaffing and abuses of power in the entrenched hospital hierarchy. Young Cathy listened intently to the harrowing stories Jean brought home from her shifts. This was the 1950s, before universal health coverage, so patients who were unable to pay were sometimes refused care, even when extremely ill. Then, as now, nurses were often stretched to the limit of their capabilities. It wasn't unheard of for two nurses to be assigned to fifty patients.

Cathy's first jobs were in the cardiology step-down unit at a major Toronto hospital. By the early 1980s, Cathy had a husband doing doctoral work and a young child. Wanting to get away from the unpredictable grind of shift work, she took a position at a private clinic on Bay Street, in the heart of Canada's corporate and banking world. At the time, Ontario was flirting with the privatization of healthcare. Extra billing was permitted for everything, and doctors at the clinic were fully on board, sending their cherry-picked young, white, and mostly healthy executive patients for lots of mostly unnecessary tests. For Cathy, the experience was profoundly disillusioning. This wasn't accessible, equitable healthcare. This was profit over people.

She applied to an advertisement for a community nurse position at the community health centre in leafy Riverdale, which at the time had a strong working-class component. To her delight, she was hired. The clinic staff later told her they had been impressed by the fact that she walked around the neighbourhood before the interview to get a feel for it and its residents. Sometimes it's the simple, human things you do that count the most.

All the clinic's doctors were on salary, so patients were treated equitably. The dynamic was communal. The team not only mentored Cathy but also involved her in all aspects of patient care. In *Knapsack*, she writes, "It was in that clinic where I truly learned that health is political, the personal is political and that politics is the most important determinant of health." It was also where she learned what it meant to be responsive to community needs, and to use advocacy for health promotion. Later, when she was working at Street Health, an independent nursing clinic for unhoused people, Cathy learned that securing housing for homeless patients meant they wouldn't need to be treated on the streets. Crowded shelters led to outbreaks of infectious diseases, and years of homelessness took a great toll on people's health and longevity.

She also learned that many of the stereotypes she had held about homeless people were dead wrong. Each person had a story, and skills, that were uniquely their own (one patient would play Beethoven on the clinic's piano; another shared anecdotes about working on the Sky-Dome). She learned that being homeless didn't necessarily mean living on the street. In Toronto, still ground zero for the homelessness crisis in Canada, 7,000 people were in shelters, many of them families with children. By 2023, that number had grown to over 10,000.

In 1982, Cathy left the Riverdale clinic to return to nursing school. She had a diploma, not a degree, which wouldn't get her where she wanted professionally. She graduated with honours and received several awards.

When she returned to work as a nurse practitioner at community-based clinics, she was disappointed to find the scope of her practice was highly dependent on the whims of whichever doctor happened to be in charge. It created a kind of cognitive dissonance. While some doctors trusted her and gave her free rein, others treated her like their personal assistant. And when she later voiced her desire to do a master's degree, management wouldn't accommodate her, even though she was willing to do it part-time on a reduced salary.

Her desire to make a difference and to use her nursing degree to its full capacity eventually landed her at Street Health, a non-profit, community-based and nursing-led organization at Sherbourne and Dundas, the epicentre of Toronto's homelessness disaster. The clinic used a primary healthcare model, which meant that staff went out to the community where the unhoused were, and held nursing clinics in drop-ins and shelters. Over time, her work as a street nurse would take her way beyond the drop-ins and shelters into parks and alleyways, and under bridges to squatters' camps.

It became clear to Cathy early on that bandages and pills only went so far when it came to treating her clients. To find real health solutions, she'd have to go further upstream to the source of their problems, which in most cases was the simple fact that they didn't have a roof over their heads or a stable home life to shield them from factors like violence and disease, which could damage their health.

Health is influenced by many factors, including a person's genetics, age, and behaviour. But it also has powerful social determinants, which, unlike genetics or age, can be positively affected by interventions from lawmakers and other public officials. This convinced Cathy that advocacy work is nursing work. Smoking affects life expectancy, but so does living on the street or in a crowded shelter with a tuberculosis, SARS, or Covid outbreak.

Cathy already had a strong social awareness influenced by the disarmament and feminist movements of the Cold War 1980s. The work of Australian anti-nuclear activist and pediatrician Helen Caldicott inspired Cathy to become involved in the Canadian peace movement and to draft a resolution for multilateral disarmament at the Registered Nurses of Ontario (RNAO) annual meeting. That same decade, she co-founded the highly influential Nurses for Social Responsibility (NSR), whose mandate was to advocate for "the elimination of inequality, oppression, violence, and aggression." The NSR collaborated with likeminded groups to fight for women's rights and related issues like pay equity. It also lobbied against a proposed bylaw to prohibit begging in tourist areas and for the establishment of freestanding abortion clinics and AIDS hospices, both of which were controversial at the time (sadly, the former have become newly controversial. The threat of nuclear war having obvious relevance to nursing, the NSR also tackled military issues, warning the public about dangers like the potential health impacts of the Gulf War.

Cathy's commitment to these causes has gotten her arrested on multiple occasions: for protesting militarism at a Toronto weapons plant and the Ministry of Defence in Ottawa, homelessness in Ontario at Queen's Park, the G7 Summit in Toronto, and apartheid at South Africa's embassy in Ottawa.

Some of her battles are less obviously connected to the social determinants of health, like the fight to maintain the long-form census, an invaluable source of data about trends in vulnerable populations and thus a crucial tool for social advocacy (unfortunately, on this front the NSR suffered a rare failure).

Cathy's goals haven't always aligned with those of mainstream nursing organizations. In the mid 1980s she lobbied against the return of the death penalty, an issue which she saw as a natural fit for nursing, like disarmament. How could a profession whose mandate was saving lives support the officially sanctioned taking of one? But while various other professional associations joined the NSR's coalition on the issue, the CNA declined.

The late 1990s, when Mike Harris was premier of Ontario, were particularly dark times for healthcare. In response to an alarming rise in discriminatory treatment of homeless people, including police brutality and hate crimes—one homeless woman had her mouth taped shut with a dirty bandage in an ER—Cathy co-founded the Street Nurses Network (SNN), a grassroots network of nurses from across the city who worked with homeless and underhoused clients in a variety of settings: primary care clinics, shelters, parishes, and needle-exchange sites.

Although Harris was out of power by the early 2000s, the damage was done. Problems related to homelessness weren't going away; if anything, they were getting worse. Tensions and crowding led to unhoused people getting barred from health centres and shelters, and unhealthy conditions led to outbreaks of Norwalk virus and, shockingly, tuberculosis. This was a particularly intense time for Cathy. She secured flu shots for people in rooming houses, tackled a bedbug epidemic, campaigned to stop the use of a toxic lice treatment, and launched an action group to secure an inquest into tuberculosis deaths, which won better public health monitoring. She got media savvy. Long before everyone had one in their pocket, she started carrying a camera to document what she saw, which amounted to refugee-level conditions in what was supposed to be a developed country. She sought and found allies who were reporters and learned how to strategically leak a story.

By 2004, *advocacy* had become a dirty word in some circles. Fearful of funding cuts, social and health organizations effectively imposed a code of silence on their employees. Cathy and her colleagues were forbidden from attending rallies or speaking publicly about anything that could be construed as political. Minutes of meetings were scanned for anti-government sentiment. This posed a conundrum for Cathy: how could she continue to be a nurse if, in her view, nursing and activism were inseparable?

Her solution, as always, was to fight on. The year 1998 saw one of her greatest triumphs when the Toronto Disaster Relief Committee declared homelessness a national emergency. This immediately resulted in a federal program to tackle homelessness and laid the groundwork for the resuscitation of the national housing program, which built 20,000 units a year. (The co-op housing where Cathy lives, in a mixed-income community near Toronto's St. Lawrence Market, was built as part of this program.)

In 1999, when a sprawling tent city sprang up on land known to be polluted with heavy metals, Cathy worked with the Toronto Disaster Relief Committee to alleviate conditions. Tents were replaced with pre-fab housing; flimsy makeshift shelters were insulated and roofs were augmented. Wood stoves, portable toilets, and, at one point, even generators and running water were brought in. Someone tipped Cathy off that residents were going to be evicted, and she managed to get there, with cameras, before the police arrived. The international attention that ensued (the area in question would have been the site of the Olympic athletes' village if Toronto had won its bid for the Games) ultimately helped to secure a housing pilot program for evictees.

Despite such victories, Cathy believes things are worse than ever. In the years leading up to the pandemic, she was a thorn in the side of Toronto mayor John Tory, drawing attention to his failure to build suitable and affordable housing for the homeless (as promised) and his resistance to acknowledging homelessness as an emergency. She was highly critical, too, of the strong-arm tactics of Toronto Police in handling the encampment evictions. (When we talked to her on the podcast in April 2021, her focus was on speeding up vaccinations in the encampments and in shelter hotels.)

On the positive side, Cathy was impressed by the number of physicians who stepped up to talk publicly about healthcare and social justice during Covid. One was Dr. Naheed Dosani, a physician advocate who came to Canada as a refugee from Uganda in the 1970s and started Palliative Education and Care for the Homeless (PEACH). This program brings together housing, mental health, and healthcare professionals to provide community-based hospice palliative care for the unhoused. Like Cathy, Dr. Dosani uses his large online presence to try to destigmatize homelessness and effect change.

She has fewer positive things to say about the nursing community as a whole, which she once described as "frozen in a cryogenic sleep, unaware of current political affairs and modern issues and how they relate to the practice of nursing." Many of Cathy's nursing heroes are figures from the past. Like Marion Dewar, a nurse activist and Ottawa mayor who challenged Canadian cities to bring Vietnamese boat people to the country in the 1970s. Cathy wants to see more nurses on the front lines, not just of care, but of social justice. She's aware that, given the still-entrenched hierarchies of healthcare, many nurses fear losing their jobs if they speak out. In fact, she believes she herself was blacklisted due to her activism. For several years in the 2010s, she had difficulty finding work.

CATHY CONTINUES TO identify as a street nurse, although she gave up her active nursing licence in 2022 to protest Ontario premier Doug Ford's treatment of nurses. Self-employed, today she is a visiting practitioner in the department of politics and public administration at Toronto Metropolitan University, working with students and faculty on housing, homelessness, and advocacy. Ironically, when the university president created the position for her, the nursing school did not offer to host her in their department. The politics department grabbed her instead.

Although medical education has changed dramatically, Cathy laments that most nursing curricula still don't include political and economic theory or discussion of racism and classism. The "disaster walks" she began years ago to show politicians and others the gravity of the homelessness problem in their own backyards have morphed into community health and social justice walks with students. She takes the lessons to the street—to City Hall, inner-city communities like Regent Park, grocery stores, and activist group meetings and rallies. Along the way, she'll ask the students who their city councillor, MPP, or MP is. Sadly, most of them don't know.

Still, for many students, the walks and Cathy's teaching are eye-opening, life-changing experiences. At minimum, they expand awareness of what a nurse can do. There's an army of Cathy Crowe protégés out there, and it's growing.

With the death rate of homeless people inside city shelters unacceptably high—something she calls "social murder"—one of Cathy's major life goals remains restoring Canada's national housing program.

Originally put in place in response to a housing crisis, and highlighted by protests of returning WWII veterans, the highly successful program was cancelled in 1993. In 2017, Justin Trudeau's Liberal government announced a national housing *strategy* based on human rights. Close, but no cigar.

A lot of Cathy's work took place before social media, when getting the word out meant summoning a reporter and a cameraperson. Today, she tweets and retweets constantly about the issues she's passionate about: homelessness, social justice, Indigenous rights, fair working conditions for nurses—plus Blue Jays baseball and Canadian art. In April 2021, when Canadian federal Finance Minister Chrystia Freeland posted a picture of the new high-heeled shoes she bought to present the federal budget (a long-held tradition), Cathy, in typical form, replied by posting a picture of one of her homeless patient's shoes (let's just say they weren't new or shiny).

Cathy backs political candidates with progressive positions and gives kudos when they're deserved. But if a post is factually incorrect, she immediately calls bull. "This Tweet is no longer available" is a common sight above one of Cathy's takedowns.

She's a collector of political buttons and, maybe a bit surprisingly, Harlequin romance nursing books. She's also a huge film buff. For years she's attended the Toronto International Film Festival, taking in twenty to thirty movies over ten days (the chapters in *Knapsack* are all themed around her favourite films). She's made several documentaries and is even featured in one: Shelley Saywell's *Street Nurse* (2002), which often gets screened at Canadian nursing colleges.

Nursing school taught us about pathology, disease, microbiology. No one talked or thought critically about the systemic causes of poor health. Thanks to Cathy, a new generation of nurses is learning that we need to advocate for things to move forward. But of course, her message isn't just for nurses. It's for everyone.

Amie

I *got good at* holding my bladder in nursing school. A little *too* good. The habit continued into my career as a labour and delivery nurse. Sometimes I'd go an entire 12-hour shift without peeing or drinking water for the simple reason that I didn't have time to.

But my party trick became a liability when I started developing kidney stones. For those lucky enough never to have had them, kidney stones form when the minerals and salts naturally present in urine become concentrated and hardened. Stones that stay small and don't leave the kidney are generally benign. Problems usually start when small stones grow into large ones and travel down the tiny tube between the kidney and the bladder called the ureter, where they become stuck and block urine flow. If you need to pee but find when you get to the toilet that almost nothing comes out, and then a few minutes later you need to pee again, that's a pretty good sign that you've got kidney stones.

The pain of kidney stones is intense and, like all pain, hard to describe. A lot of mothers who have had them swear the process of passing them is worse than childbirth. My own three births were C-sections, so I can't speak to the accuracy of this, but kidney stones are definitely the most painful thing I've ever experienced. The sensation is something like a watermelon passing through a straw . . . in your own body.

On one of the multiple occasions when I had kidney stones, the pain became so overwhelming that I started to black out. Luckily, I was home at the time with my husband, Jordan, who called 911. As I faded in and out of consciousness, I heard him telling the medics I was a nurse, and that I had diagnosed myself with kidney stones. Prior to my first blackout, I'd done two sets of vitals on myself (heart rate, BP, response rate), got all my meds ready for the paramedics, and re-briefed Jordan on my health history, even though he obviously knew a lot of it already. We nurses will do this as a kind of courtesy to take the burden off the healthcare providers treating us (weird, right?).

When the medics arrived, I was on the toilet, pants around my ankles. Asked to rate my pain on a scale of ten, I managed to blurt out "Ten!" before promptly passing out again.

With kidney stones there's really nothing you can do beyond pain management, so they took me to the hospital, where they put me on a cocktail of IV of morphine, Toradol, and Gravol while I waited eight hours for the stone to pass. (Jordan told me later that when I came to I critiqued the EMS's IV technique, though I have no memory of this.) The process is kind of like childbirth, but without the bonus of getting a baby at the end. I'll never forget that it was Valentine's Day because when the stone finally passed the doctor came in and told me, with some amazement, that it was heart-shaped. My own feelings were less of amazement than relief. The bizarre thing about passing a kidney stone is that the pain doesn't slowly ebb away, it just . . . stops. And then you're fine.

The kidney stone experience is just one of many times I've had the healthcare tables turned on me over the years. I've also been hospitalized for a car accident, congestive heart failure, hernia repair surgery, two Caesarean sections, an ectopic pregnancy, a cystoscopy (a procedure in which the bladder is examined using a tiny camera) for gross hematuria (blood in the urine), and knee surgery. Good times! Like many nurses, I went into the profession because I wanted to help others, so being on the other side of the caregiver-patient equation hasn't always been comfortable.

This leads to the biggest conundrum nurses face when we're admitted into care: whether to disclose the fact that we're nurses. It's kind of a double-edged sword. On the one hand, not disclosing you're a nurse might come off as . . . weird? Especially if your caregivers eventually find out. On the other, admitting you're a nurse might seem like you're signalling, Hey, I know all the protocols and I've got eyes on you! Or even that you expect preferential treatment of some kind. You want *your* nurse—especially if they're new or a student—to be able to do their job without feeling intimidated or pressured (I've seen nurses so nervous sweat was dripping from their foreheads). On the flip side, sometimes instead of being nervous or super nice they become defensive. That's when things can get *really* awkward.

When I was hospitalized, I'd sometimes take out my own IV or get my own water. Why would I wait for a nurse to do something I could do perfectly well myself? Admittedly, there have been times when I worried too much about how I came across. When I was pregnant with my twins, for example, they brought me morphine, which I wasn't going to take (it makes me dizzy and nauseous). But instead of explaining this and handing back the pills—which might make me look like a "difficult" patient—I hid them under my pillow!

It's not that disclosing hasn't come in handy. During my battles with kidney stones, the hospital started discharging me with morphine tablets. I can't say for sure, but I don't think this is something they would have done for a non-nurse (and of course I didn't even take them). I've disclosed near the end of a visit just to speed up my discharge and relieve the nurse of their duty. And I usually do so when the issue concerns my kids, or if I'm 100 percent certain that the care I am receiving is inadequate. In other words, if my health or the health of my children is potentially at risk.

My concerns about self-disclosing aren't entirely based on my own experiences as a nurse treating other nurses. The three or four times this happened, my tendency was to turn up the TLC. Knowing there's a mutual understanding based on shared experience allows us to skip the preamble and get right to the care.

We don't usually admit it to outsiders, but there's a surprising amount of agreement among nurses about which professionals make the worst patients. You probably won't be surprised when I tell you that many are physicians. My reluctance about self-disclosure is shared by most nurses I know, but it doesn't seem to be shared by most doctors, many of whom will do everything they can to signal their status. Some will show up wearing their hospital badges. Others will lay it right out there: "Hi, I'm Dr. X, an *endocrinologist* from the fifth floor." Needless to say, a certain sense of entitlement usually accompanies this approach.

Other professionals who can be, well, challenging to treat—engineers, lawyers, and teachers—might be more of a surprise. They present a challenge because they are accustomed to asking questions. *Lots* of questions. And some want the answers reiterated six or seven times. Teachers always seem to arrive in the maternity ward in clusters during the summer, presumably because they schedule their births for the months when they're off work.

Engineers are the worst. They want detailed technical explanations of what's happening, then use your response as an excuse to lecture you about science and health. Once, a patient's spouse (an engineer) asked me how oxytocin is used. It's a common question, and I answered it the way I always do. His wife seemed satisfied with my explanation, but he bombarded me with aggressive questions: How exactly does it affect the baby? Where are the studies that prove it's safe? I was like, Hold on, dude . . . the internet is working and here's the doctor!

A lot of people think that because we work in healthcare, nurses must take good care of our own health and wellbeing. But this isn't the case at all. In fact, most nurses I know, me included, tend to wait a long time before getting treated, which means we're among the *sickest* patients. We let ourselves get run ragged, don't drink enough water, and ignore the signs of dehydration during shifts. (My kidney stones are a good example: I had no doubt about what was causing all the pain; I was just putting off the inevitable.) There are multiple reasons why nurses do this, but the main one is that we're really, really busy. The other reason is temperament. It's in our DNA to care for others; we don't expect others to take care of us. When nurses become patients, Murphy's Law seems to apply: everything that could go wrong *does* go wrong. Many times, my healthcare providers have asked me, "Why on earth didn't you come here sooner?"

Another common misconception about nurses is that we have insider access to better health information. The truth is that our symptoms get missed as often as they do with anyone else. The postpartum preeclampsia I experienced after the birth of my first child, for example, initially got missed. My legs had swelled to a degree I knew was unusual, but my doctor assured me the swelling would soon go down and sent me home. It didn't, and I ended up hospitalized. Even then, the nurses and doctors kept trying to discharge me, despite the fact that I was having difficulty breathing and was at risk for a pulmonary embolism, a leading cause of death among Black women post-childbirth. (Contributing to the disproportionate mortality rate for Black women in childbirth and postpartum is the fact that, due to systemic racism, our pain is often not believed, or is minimized.)

The advice I got in 2022 about surgery to repair my MPFL, the ligament that holds the kneecap in place, wasn't great either. At the time, the pandemic was still lingering, so there was a lot of fear about using a general anaesthetic, which involves intubation that opens the patient's airway, potentially exposing them and those around them to the Covid-19 virus.

Because of this, it was strongly suggested that I opt for a spinal block, which is similar to an epidural used on women during childbirth. I was told that because I would be more conscious during surgery, the spinal block would allow me to bounce back faster than general anaesthetic (it's also easier to put people to sleep than to wake them up).

Wrong again! Not only did I fall asleep during the procedure (though I was breathing on my own), but the spinal block, which freezes your lower body, takes a *long* time to wear off. As a result, I was in hospital longer than anticipated. My pain was also horribly managed. The painkillers they gave me upon discharge were basically the equivalent of Advil. By the time I got home they had worn off and I was screaming in agony. I couldn't get out of the car, and Jordan had to carry me inside. Every little bump felt like my leg was being torn off. The pharmacy was closed when I left, but the MDs could have given me proper meds to take home and the nurses could have helped advocate for this. I spent that night and the following morning in the worst pain of my life—worse than the kidney stone experience, which I didn't think was possible—all because of a systems issue and the lack of advocacy on my behalf.

This was not the end of the story. Before surgery, there was the issue of whether to use a donor tendon or one of my own. The disadvantage of using a donor tendon is that it's difficult to time the surgery, since the tendon itself has to come from a fresh cadaver. Donated tendons can also be rejected by your body, leading to further complications and surgeries. At the time, elective surgeries had been shut down for two years due to the pandemic, and I was told that if I used a donor I could possibly be waiting another two years. This just wasn't in the cards, since I couldn't walk without potentially falling. Feeling confident, I opted to use my own tendon. It would be faster! Less risky! The pain would be *slightly* higher, but the benefits would be worth it. Nope. The surgery was not fast. The tendon was taken from my hamstring, which meant that yet another part of my body was compromised, further lengthening my recovery period. And the pain was not slightly but *significantly* worse.

From admittance to discharge during that surgery, I never told my caregivers that I was a nurse, though I did come close at one point. I was in pain, and I asked my nurse for Tylenol or Advil. She told me it could be a while before she could get me something since the doctor on call wasn't around to give approval. The two nurses looking after me were not my original caregivers—I had had several, owing to the fact that my recovery was taking so long. Not only were these nurses unsympathetic, they seemed annoyed because I "wasn't really their patient." They didn't want to call the doctor for more effective pain meds, likely because they didn't want to get yelled at, given a culture that strongly dissuades nurses from calling doctors during night shifts, and because they knew I would soon be discharged. They should have advocated for me, but they chose not to.

The nurse card was between the tips of my fingers, but I held it back. (Knowing what I do now about pain management and Black patients, I would never let myself be put in a situation like that again. I've learned to always speak out and advocate for myself.) Instead, I stewed, wondering why we weren't yet at the point where something as simple as getting an over-the-counter pain medication, which I could have bought downstairs in the pharmacy, wasn't part of the chart, or readily available.

During my recovery, I decided that if I were ever in that situation again, I would self-disclose. Would they have taken me more seriously, been more likely to call the MD, if they knew I was a nurse too? I can't say for sure, but I am confident that it couldn't have made things any worse.

The whole experience drove home the importance of advocating for yourself in the healthcare system, whether you're a nurse or not. Despite what caregivers may want to believe, the patient is the one who knows themself, and their health, best.

Sara

A mie and I agree on many things, but night shifts is not one of them. I always loathed working nights. Not that I had a say in the matter. Every nurse has to do them. When you work full-time for a unionized hospital, you're just handed a schedule, which usually divides your shifts roughly into half days and half nights.

Unless you have a medical exemption, the only way to get around night shifts is to switch with someone who is working days, which I used to do as often as I could. While it's not possible to work only day shifts, you can choose to work only night shifts if you want. (This tells you how popular they are.)

Night shifts feel like a totally different world, even if it's the same unit where you work during the day. You never see management or the support staff that buzz around during the day—social workers, housekeeping, lactation consultations. It's very bare bones.

And it's much, much quieter. The patients generally aren't wandering the halls looking for conversation; they're trying to sleep. Often there are no visitors. In some hospitals visiting ends at 8 p.m., although this has been changing lately. On medical-surgical and mental health wards, nurses usually take on a higher patient load, which is normally fine since patients are usually sleeping. But the postpartum unit, where I've spent most of my working life, is different. A woman can go into labour at any hour of the night, and babies require just as much care and feeding since they're not yet on a schedule. So even though the nurse-to-patient ratio is the same as on the day shift, the lack of support staff at night makes the job harder. We have to get by without social workers, housekeepers, porters (to transport patients, take things to/from the lab), clerical support (to answer phones or put together charts), management (to help handle difficult situations), and even physicians (many are on call, either sleeping in another part of the hospital or off-site, and don't want to be disturbed unless it's an emergency).

The most challenging thing about nights was figuring out a good eating and sleeping schedule. I'd find myself eating all day and then snacking all night. Some nurses wouldn't eat at all during a night shift; I have no idea how they did it. Regardless of what or how much I ate in the day, I always felt hungry at night—starving, actually! And because you're constantly flip-flopping between night and day shifts, your body is always trying to get back to a semblance of normalcy. After a red-eye flight, most people will sleep the next day to compensate for it, but we don't have that option. Some nurses use ear plugs or sleeping pills to get enough rest after a shift, but many find they become reliant on them. After their night shifts, most nurses nap only a couple of hours so they can be on the same schedule as the rest of society. I had a co-worker who drove into a ditch when she fell asleep at the wheel after a night shift. Luckily, she got away with minor cuts and bruises; more importantly, no one else was injured. Incidents like this are more common than people realize.

A lot of nurses who have children at home actually prefer night shifts because they can sleep while the kids are at school. A nurse who trained me in my final year of school had a fifteen-year-old son who thought she slept during the night shift. It just goes to show what little awareness people can have!

Of course, the model falls apart on weekends when kids are home, or if you're a single parent. Many of us don't live in huge houses, so it's impossible not to hear what's going on outside the bedroom door.

When I worked night shifts regularly, some people didn't understand why I couldn't do things during the day. If I did decide to undertake an activity—run errands, go to appointments, or attend any kind of social event—I'd have to sacrifice part of my "night" or just lose out on sleep entirely. Imagine asking a friend to meet you for lunch at 3 a.m. and being surprised when they turn you down.

As Amie has noted, night shifts have their own unique culture. This includes sleep breaks, which are not in our collective agreement. Sleep breaks are a bit like nursing fight club: the first rule is that no one talks about them, at least not outside the unit, and especially not in front of your manager, even though most managers used to be nurses, so they know!

So why *don't* we talk about them? I suppose it's because it would seem like the mice were taking advantage of the cats being away. A lot of nurses (I'm looking at you, Amie!) deliberately work nights to get away from management. But it's not like we prioritize sleep breaks above our patients' health and safety. The reality is the opposite. A nurse is going to be much better able to cope with an emergency if they're well rested, not burning the midnight oil waiting for the worst to happen. Call it Murphy's Law, but most of the true emergencies I've experienced as a nurse have happened at night.

I've been on units where nobody slept. Instead, we'd make popcorn and watch a movie together in the break room. I've also worked on units where maybe half the staff slept while the other half read a book, listened to music, or ordered food from the huge binders of takeout menus we kept (these being the days before online delivery services). Many of the deliverers came to know us by name. Another hospital where I worked had a 24-hour gym, and some nurses actually worked out in the middle of the night!

But I always preferred the units where breaks were imposed. I love sleep, and I find it really hard to ignore when my body screams at me to shut everything down. Still, no matter how you approach them, night shifts wreak havoc with your body in a way that will eventually catch up with you.

The way sleep breaks work depends on the hospital. On one unit, the charge nurse orchestrated breaks by making a list of available rooms, then telling you, military-style, where and when you were going. I actually liked this approach because it meant I didn't have to use the limited energy I had at night to think about how, or where, to spend my break. Other units used a first-come, first-served approach. Then there were units that operated by seniority, with the longest-serving nurses getting first-pick of break time and place.

That was the way it worked in the NICU, which had a huge staff. Because I was relatively junior, I sometimes had to "make" a bed by putting two chairs together. Our break room had three very coveted couches. Staff would race there to secure a couch by pinning a note to it bearing their scrawled name. It was a bit of a game of musical chairs. When I was the loser of the game, I sometimes ended up just walking the ward halls. To avoid competition, some nurses sought out empty rooms on other floors where they could sneak away to sleep.

The longest breaks I ever had—three hours!—were on an ante-natal and post-natal high-risk unit where I worked briefly due to short staffing. On my first shift, I was scheduled for a 3 to 6 a.m. break. However, I was anxious to get a jump start on my tasks, which including weighing and doing bloodwork on three babies before the doctors arrived at 7:30 a.m., so I decided to go back to the floor early. I knew they'd be annoyed if everything wasn't ready on their patients' charts, and I was worried that an hour and a half wouldn't be enough time to finish everything I needed to do.

But when I showed up at the nursing station, the charge nurse gave me a stern look and shook her head: I *had* to stay on break until 6 a.m! I didn't feel I was in a position to argue, so I made my way back to the cold, dark room at the end of the hall—in keeping with my low position on the ward hierarchy—and lay there staring at the ceiling until the appointed hour.

The unofficial aspect of sleep breaks sometimes made for awkward situations. I remember one night a nurse was assigned to a room that was suddenly needed for an incoming patient. When I knocked on the door to warn her she didn't respond, so I had to go in and shake her awake. Completely disoriented, she jumped off the bed and ran out of the room as the patient was rolling down the hall towards her!

The night shift isn't always the calm oasis people might imagine. One night while I was walking down the unit hall, I heard a thumping coming from a nearby room. I poked my head in and saw a strange, rhythmic movement happening behind the curtain of the bed at the far end of the room. I walked past three patients who seemed oblivious to what was going on and pulled back the curtain. A woman who had given birth a few hours earlier was seated in a chair in full seizure mode, convulsing and drooling, her eyes rolled back in her head. The scene was made more frightening because her newborn, whom she had obviously been feeding, was still on her lap. I moved the baby to the bed and called a Code Blue. (I learned later that the mom was on meds for epilepsy; the sleep deprivation and altered routine of childbirth had likely triggered the seizure.)

In the postpartum unit we rarely had a Code Blue, which usually means someone's heart has stopped beating. Add to this the fact that most of the nurses responding to the Code Blue were on sleep break, so they were pretty disoriented when they came streaming into the room. But the adrenaline of the emergency quickly dispelled that fog, and everyone was soon pitching in doing what needed to be done.

It was afterwards, while we were stabilizing the patient—who was mortified by the whole experience—when someone yelled, "Where's the baby?!"

For a split second we all panicked and looked around. Then someone else called out "I have it!" At some point during all the mayhem, a nurse had removed the baby from the bed and handed it to one of the dads in the room, although no one could remember doing so.

After working a night shift I would head, bleary eyed, onto the subway, a single person walking against the sea of commuters rushing in the opposite direction to their daytime jobs. I'd try my hardest not to fall asleep on the way home. Sometimes I didn't have the energy to even shower. Or I'd worry that a shower would wake me up when I needed to sleep.

Then came my favourite part of a night shift: the moment when, after pulling down the blackout blinds and putting on some white noise, I could finally close my eyes and drift off to sleep. If I was lucky, I'd wake up refreshed. But if one of these factors didn't align and I didn't have a good sleep, I'd wake up disoriented and have to repeat the process all over again. Nights will do that to you.

NURSE WITH GRIT

Alyce Faye Wattleton (b. 1943)

The Missouri-born only child of a construction worker father and travelling preacher mother, Alyce Faye Wattleton worked as a public health nurse and nurse-midwife before becoming the youngest person and first African American woman (as well as the first woman since Margaret Sanger) to serve as president of the Planned Parenthood Federation of America (PPFA) in 1978. Having seen firsthand the life-threatening effects of unsafe, illegal abortions, Wattleton spent much of her fourteen years at PPFA battling the socially conservative administrations of Ronald Reagan and George Bush in their attempts to restrict legal abortion. Other successes included securing federal funding for birth control and prenatal programs, and the legalization of the sale of mifepristone, a medication used to terminate pregnancies. After leaving the PPFA, Wattleton went on to host a talk show. She created a non-profit think tank, the Center for the Advancement of Women, whose goal was "dismantling the obstacles that impede full equality for women." In addition to a long list of awards, including the Women's Honors in Public Service from the American Nurses Association, Wattleton holds at least fifteen honorary doctoral degrees.

Natalie Stake-Doucet

Patient advocacy is an official job that comes naturally to most nurses. And because we're not paid piecemeal for our work—unlike doctors, we don't have financial incentives to change the way we practise (we don't get more money, for example, if we give a patient a bath instead of a shower)—in most cases our hearts are in the right place.

Given the built-in power differential between doctors and nurses, there are times when patient advocacy can get tricky. Our main superpower in that regard isn't sexy: it's paperwork. We document *eeeeverything*. Everyone knows the mantra of real estate: location, location, location. In nursing it's: document, document, document.

But advocating for ourselves and one another? Not so much. As a profession, we have had an unfortunate tendency to stick our heads in the sand and leave the advocating to others, especially when there's a political dimension to it. People like Cathy Crowe are unfortunately the exception, not the rule.

But with global working conditions deteriorating to crisis levels since the pandemic, it's no exaggeration to say that self-advocacy has become crucial to our survival (and by extension, the survival of the healthcare system). Part of our mission with the podcast, and with this book, is to highlight inspiring nurses who are leading the way, the ones who are making a difference to the profession through advocacy.

A name that stands out in this area is Natalie Stake-Doucet, past president and spokesperson of the Quebec Nurses Association and associate professor at Université de Montreal. You might say that advocacy and social justice are in Natalie's blood. She began her career as an RN in 2010 in a rural hospital and later moved to Montreal to specialize in mental health and forensic psychiatry. She was a babe in arms when her flower-power hippie parents started taking her to protests. (Her American mother is a feminist who crusaded against the war in Vietnam; her French-Canadian father is a long-time social justice activist.) A lot of kids would be bored walking along the street chanting slogans, but not Natalie. She loved the energy, the noise, the colour.

Later, when she became a nurse and started grappling with the issues facing the profession, falling into an advocacy role felt entirely natural. Natalie will often say of nursing that it's one of the best jobs performed in some of the worst conditions.

She also believes that, in their role as caregivers, nurses have a unique perspective on the human condition and the way social problems directly impact health. Change nursing, and you can help change the world.

In 2020, Natalie put her doctoral studies on hold mid-pandemic so she could assist in the trenches of long-term care (LTC), which were being hit hard. As part of a coalition of patient advocates, family MDs, social workers, and others, she helped produce a policy brief for the provincial government explaining the threat the pandemic posed to LTC, based on what other countries had experienced.

When the government failed to respond, the coalition took a new tack. They sent their brief to the provincial opposition party and wrote editorials that got published in the media. The LTC home where Natalie was working during this period was the worst hit in the province. Fifty percent of the staff and 80 percent of the residents developed Covid-19 (half of the residents eventually died). Walking into the facility was like entering a portal into a dystopian alternate reality. In April 2020, Natalie started keeping a public diary on Facebook. It was a way to process the trauma, but it also brought attention to the apocalypse playing out in real time. Some of her posts received thousands of shares. An artist named Jenny Cartwright made an audio documentary based on the diary. It later won the Prix Numix award.

But awareness didn't reduce the deaths. Part of the problem was the provincial healthcare system's bureaucracy, which was too inflexible to rise to the occasion and provide crucial supplies like personal protection equipment (PPE). To get the protection they needed, Natalie and her co-workers would have to be even more creative.

Then an unexpected opportunity arose, and the nurses seized it. The provincial minister of health had just concluded a press conference in which she declared that PPE supply was not an issue. Five minutes later, Natalie's nursing coordinator walked in and said there were no more protective gowns available. Nurses had the option of washing the ones they had or wearing patient gowns, which were short-sleeved and also in very short supply. No one had any idea where to get more equipment. It wasn't even clear who was in charge of procuring it.

The coordinator repeated that if Natalie and her colleagues wanted more gowns they would "just have to do laundry." (This was particularly galling, given that the nurses were trying to keep patients from dying while grotesquely understaffed. She said later, "I felt the sexism of that assumption in my bones." A few days earlier, Natalie had heard the minister address healthcare workers through the media. She had actually said, "If you're missing anything, call me."

Natalie decided to do just that. Directly after her shift, she called the minister's office. The assistant, who was confused, put her off.

Faced with the same lack of PPE, nurses in New York City had been posting images of themselves on social media dressed in garbage bags. One of Natalie's colleagues, an orderly and fellow troublemaker—as Natalie often refers to herself—decided to do the same thing.

It was shortly after a journalist wrote "Can I call you?" in the comments under the photo of the orderly in the garbage bag that the first gowns started appearing on Natalie's ward, as if by magic. This, even as the administration threatened the orderly, telling her she would "pay" for her post.

Undeterred, Natalie and her colleagues worked to build a network of solidarity that would allow them to bypass the slow-moving healthcare system. "Shit got done," she said. "To me, that's the most beautiful thing to come out of it . . . no matter how harrowing it was, it showed that the true face of healthcare is us. We're the ones carrying it on our shoulders, literally."

When facilities and businesses offered to donate PPE in small quantities Natalie thought the government would probably not bother with, she picked up the donations herself by bicycle and delivered them to supervised injection sites and the places that needed them the most.

And when Quebec's Ministry of Health suspended all collective agreements during the pandemic, nurses staged sit-in strikes, each of which led to some form of immediate change. None of Natalie's colleagues had a problem stepping up when this was required. But a year into the suspension, many felt they were being taken advantage of. They were often called in on a moment's notice, for example, to deal with what amounted to non-emergency, run-of-the-mill staffing issues. Part-time nurses were forced to come in full-time or to work untenable schedules, even in facilities that hadn't had a single Covid case. (A quarter of all Covid cases in Quebec were among healthcare workers.)

There was a phenomenal quantity of forced overtime, which was particularly challenging for nurses with young children.

Natalie believes that the top-down, military healthcare model that has been in place since the Nightingale era works against nurses by making them feel their place is at the bottom of the heap. She wants this to change. She also wants nurses to raise one another up more and "to see their worth collectively, so we can collectively say F-you to the forces that try to keep us down." Working towards this, she routinely encourages colleagues to get to know one another, to figure out the most pressing issues at work and see what can be done about them. She wants nurses to be less afraid of conflict and of questioning authority, to be confident that in the long run, they'll gain more than they lose. (As an example, she uses her family members, who debate fiercely all the time yet remain close.)

"While there is a risk, we also have to see it as a responsibility, and also see the incredible value that our professional opinion has as nurses in the public arena when discussing issues like LTC, like the pandemic, like PPE. If we don't speak out, there's a giant piece of information that's missing. And no decision-maker is going to be able to make a proper decision if he or she doesn't have our point of view. If we all spoke out, we'd be unstoppable."

Amie

When I was still debating whether to go into nursing, I visited the website of my prospective college and clicked on "What it takes to be a nurse." The link took me to a document put out by the College of Nurses of Ontario that listed some of nursing's requisite skills. These included problem-solving skills, critical thinking, and developing and then relying on professional judgment. It all sounded great to me. I was excited by the prospect of going into a caring profession that was based on logic and science. (I glossed over the parts about putting up with noxious smells and the unpredictable behaviour of others.)

And yet a surprising number of students go into nursing unaware that it's a STEM (science, technology, engineering, mathematics) subject. Many have the notion (going back to Florence Nightingale) that nursing is an art or a calling. In my opinion, this notion has served to dilute and demean the profession over time. But more on that later.

Until about fifteen years ago, you could get a two-year nursing diploma through a local hospital. Nowadays the process is way more rigorous. By the time I got to school in 2004, you needed either a four-year Bachelor of Science degree with a nursing subspecialty from a college or university, or a straight Bachelor of Nursing degree (in the US, there are many more pathways to a nursing career, including an associate's degree). And despite the rising demand for nurses due to an aging workforce and the exodus from the profession during the pandemic, getting into nursing school is harder than it's ever been. Candidates with a 94 percent average are being turned away. I went into nursing school with my eyes wide open and was still astounded when I got the course list and counted the number of textbooks I had to read.

The workload and the newness of it all meant that first year was by far the most difficult and gruelling period. Even the "bird" courses we had to take were designed to be more challenging than necessary; they required essays when multiple-choice tests would have sufficed. The focus of these courses were the fluffy, spiritual-sounding "theories of caring" fashioned by Florence Nightingale and Jean Watson (as far as I'm aware, there are no equivalent models or theories in medical school). Watson's theory of "authentic presence," for example, involved "enabling and sustaining the deep belief system and subjective life-world of self and one being cared for." If nursing is a calling, then I call BS.

In addition to these theories, and to help us better understand our mission as nurses, we were made to study so-called "care frameworks." These were often presented in the form of colourful graphs with arrows. Feeding patients wasn't just a way to provide nutrition, it promoted socialization! Taking them for walks didn't just restore mobility, it built trust! And we should be sure to smile when doing these things! The illustrations of happy, relaxed-looking nurses that accompanied care frameworks left the impression that I'd be spending a lot of my day as a nurse bonding with patients one-on-one. But the typical nurse-patient ratio in hospitals is around 1:7, and in some places, the ratio is lower.

What bothered me the most was the certainty that a caring, empathetic person couldn't be "created" just by taking a course. You're either compassionate or you're not. There's no objective proof of the "mean-girl-to-nurse pipeline"—the theory, hotly debated on Reddit and TikTok, that mean girls in high school disproportionately end up being nurses—but anecdotally speaking, it often felt like it. I met characters in nursing school that I wouldn't want touching or caring for me. I also encountered great nurses who were terrible colleagues.

From Nurse Ratched in *One Flew Over the Cuckoo's Nest* to Annie Wilkes in *Misery* to Charlotte Diesel in *High Anxiety* to Elle Driver in *Kill Bill* to the murderous nursing duo in *American Horror Story: Roanoke,* popular culture loves a nasty nurse. These characters are scary because they go against maternal stereotypes and prey upon our human fear of finding ourselves helpless and in the "care" of someone who means us harm. More frightening still, these figures exist in real life. Canadian RN and convicted serial killer Elizabeth Wettlaufer murdered eight seniors and attempted to kill six others before she finally got caught in 2016. And could there be anything creepier than "smiling nurse" Lucy Letby? In 2023 she was sentenced to life in prison for murdering seven infants in the UK (it is suspected she killed many more) and attempting to murder at least six others by injecting air and insulin into their bloodstreams. Then there's Charles Cullen, subject of Netflix's *The Good Nurse: A True Story of Medicine, Madness, and Murder.* He murdered dozens if not hundreds of patients in New Jersey over sixteen years, mostly by overdose, before his arrest in 2003.

Fortunately, your average nurse is neither a martyr, a mean girl, or a psycho. She's someone like me in that she has a passion for working with people. Nurses are genuine folks who want to help people during their lowest, most vulnerable moments and see them come out the other side better than they came in. This includes our dying patients. Helping someone achieve a dignified death by going through the stages with them makes it worth all the blood, sweat, and tears.

IN OUR SECOND term we learned to do head-to-toe assessments and started our clinicals. First-year students nearly always get put into gerontology or long-term care, and I was no different. You're not really expected to do actual nursing work in these early placements. It's more about shadowing nurses to see how they do things. (This seemed to irritate a lot of them—probably because there was no incentive for them to do it. More on this later too.) In LTC, we were expected to talk with patients and perform basic care: take them to the bathroom, wash them or change incontinence briefs, take their vitals, and get familiar with their medications. We learned to make beds, sometimes with patients in them (I started mitering the corners of our bed at home until Jordan told me to stop). Standard stuff. It was about connecting and interacting with people who were ill.

My first patient was a lovely woman with dementia named Constance. My shift was to begin at 7 a.m., and my preceptor told me to make sure I got Constance on the toilet by 7:30. I was to leave her there for approximately half an hour. It was my only task, and it should have been simple. The power of following directions! (Although now I think: "How awful to have to sit on the toilet for half an hour.")

Bright-eyed and bushy-tailed on that first morning, I was talking Constance's ear off as I brushed her teeth and combed her hair, time the furthest thing from my mind. Suddenly a shadow fell over her face. "I need to go! Hurry, dear!" She was seated on the commode but still wearing adult briefs, so I started manoeuvreing her into standing position to help get them off. As I did so, my preceptor's instructions came back to me, albeit too late. Suddenly there were feces everywhere: down Constance's legs, on her slippers and gown, on my partially gloved hands, on the floor, on the commode, and on the diaper, which I still hadn't managed to remove. It was as if a silent but deadly bomb had gone off. This was in pre-pandemic days, before it was common to wear masks, so the stench was overwhelming. Constance was embarrassed and horrified, and so was I—though I tried my best not to show it.

Residents were bathed only on alternate days. This not being a bath day, I spent over an hour attempting to clean Constance, and the mess all around us, by hand. Making a terrible situation worse was the fact that every time I wiped her, feces kept coming out. Overwhelmed by this smelly, chaotic shit-storm, I started crying.

I WAS STILL in tears when my preceptor finally walked in the room. Her reaction proved that she was a kind, amazing teacher: instead of reprimanding me for failing to follow her instructions, she put on gloves and a gown and immediately came to my aid.

The only good part about Constance having dementia was that by the time she and the room were cleaned up, she had forgotten about the entire incident. Changed and comfortable back in her sitting area, it was as if nothing had ever happened. "What's your name again, dearie?" she asked me, smiling sweetly.

I, however, did not forget so quickly. "What have I got myself into?" I remember thinking on the way home. "If this is what nursing is, I can't do it."

The next morning, I got Constance on the toilet shortly after I arrived, and the day went off without a hitch. I also made one of my first decisions about my future career: as much as I enjoyed the company and the wisdom of elderly patients, I was not going to work in long-term care.

It was during that same placement that I witnessed my first death as a care provider. My clinical preceptor had approached me and some other students and explained that the death of one of the facility's residents was imminent. Would we like to be in the room as witnesses? The man had no family. It would be a learning opportunity, and our presence might provide some comfort to him. With a solemn sense of mission, we agreed.

There were eight of us in the room—seven students plus our preceptor, who had briefly described the stages of dying to us before we entered. An ideal death is generally thought to be one in which the patient is surrounded by their loved ones. Something like my grandad's death, when we sat around singing, touching, telling stories, crying, and laughing. This environment was completely different. It made me uneasy. We were clinically observing rather than keeping vigil. It would clearly not be appropriate for us to comfort this stranger, whom we hadn't even seen when he was conscious. We did know that the man had children from whom he'd become estranged, and as much as I tried to withhold judgment, I couldn't help dwelling on this. Whatever the reason the children were not present, I still felt good knowing that our company meant the man would not die alone.

Even though I had been told it would happen, when the patient's Cheyne-Stokes breathing began I felt deeply disturbed. (I didn't recall my grandfather having Cheyne-Stokes, but I guess he must have.) We gave him scopolamine subcutaneously to clear his secretions. About half an hour later his chest stopped rising. This was startling in its finality; you could have heard a pin drop in the room. The minutes that followed were awkward. I think some of us wanted to make a kind gesture of some sort, to say something. But how could we put in a good word for this man we didn't know?

The constant presence of death in LTC made the work feel heavy. I saw nurses lose patients regularly. It was more confirmation that this was not the right environment for me. (Mostly due to my passion for true crime, I had briefly been interested in being a coroner—that is, until I picked up a coroner's manual and actually read it.) We talked a lot in class about building therapeutic relationships. It seemed even harder to imagine doing so in a place like this, where death never seemed far away. At school, we were taught to take a caring, therapeutic approach, and to "check our feelings at the door." This felt like an impossible task then, and it still does. As nurses, we grieve every loss, regardless of whether it's considered "acceptable."

I loved working with elderly patients. I loved their stories and the wisdom that they so often bestowed. But there were also things about LTC—beyond the poop—that made it feel like a bad fit for me. A major issue was the lack of regulation (which became a huge issue during the pandemic). I think this is where nurses need to get real with themselves: Don't work in clinical areas that you don't enjoy, or that you aren't mentally or physically equipped to handle. Nurses need to find the area that works best with their personality and interests and allows them to grow intellectually.

IN SECOND YEAR—probably my favourite—we got down to the business of health. We learned about the biology of disease and how to treat a patient depending on how they present, whether through wound care or IV medication. We did charting and lots of writing, learned how vital signs (heart rate, blood pressure, respiration) interact and what conditions might affect them. What I enjoyed most was the critical thinking, the sleuthing to discover what was wrong and how to correct it through nursing treatments and—this was the big one—communication. We still had to take nursing theory, which I wasn't happy about, but I mastered the art of regurgitating someone else's opinion in APA format. It felt like I now had a foundation for a practice, like I was learning the game.

When I found out I was going to be in maternal-child for second-term clinicals, it felt like I'd gotten away with something. I was going to be with *babies*?! No daily death or exploding feces (at least not in massive, adult quantities)? Bonus!

On top of doing postpartum work with mothers and babies, I got to observe a vaginal birth and a C-section. I'd never seen a baby being born, not even on TV, and I hadn't been reading the birthing section in my textbooks—not that they could have prepared me for what I saw. (I'm a "doer": I need to touch and see things to grasp them.) With the vaginal birth, I was completely taken aback that a female body could do such crazy work, that it could change shape to accommodate this gigantic football. I also thought: "I want to try this someday."

The C-section experience was very different. We hadn't talked about the OR in class yet, and as I entered the frosty room in my gown, mask, and goggles, I was full of anxiety. It felt like I was breathing into a paper bag.

The surgeon made her incision, then started digging her hands into the patient's belly. I pushed myself against the wall. Blood has a very particular smell in large quantities—one I hadn't been aware of until that moment—and it hit me hard. It's metallic, funky, earthy, and organic, a bit like the way things smell when you come back inside on a wet day . . . but not as clean. By now I was nauseous, lightheaded, and sweating. I knew that if I didn't sit down right away I would pass out, so I grabbed a nearby stool.

I and some other students had taken turns observing the surgery. Afterwards I heard one of them say what a great experience it had been. *Great* was not the word that came to my mind. I had found it amazing but overwhelming. I couldn't imagine ever getting over the cutting, or the Balfour retractor blade—a tool that was used to protect the bladder flap from being cut and sometimes used to stretch the incision. There was the blood. Sooo much blood . . . .

There were the overwhelming emotions. Patients and their partners witnessed their babies being pulled through a ten-centimetre incision in an unnatural, sterile environment (necessarily so) that was so different from that of a vaginal birth. It was too much for me at that moment. Was surgery something else I'd have to scratch from my list of professional possibilities? Maybe I can only do postpartum, I thought.

Years later, when I'd gotten over my squeamishness and was working full-time in labour and delivery, I frequently saw partners pass out. Sometimes I caught them before they hit their head on the floor. If I sensed that a partner or family member was woozy (sometimes it was super obvious; image a character in *Mortal Kombat* who exaggeratedly spins around before collapsing), I would tell them to focus on their partner's face, and by all means to avoid looking at what was happening below her chest!

As much as I loved second year, this was also the point when I started experiencing crippling anxiety. A major trigger was our in-class introduction to dosage calculations. Sometimes a medication isn't dispensed in the amount you need, so you have to calculate it based on what you've got on hand. Giving a patient an incorrect dose can severely impact or even kill them, so these calculations had to be precise. There was no room for error.

My awareness of all the possible consequences of an incorrect calculation weighed heavily on me, even though we were just practising, not doing them in a real-world setting. It felt like we'd gone from "This is fun!" to "Careful you don't kill someone!" Math had never been an issue for me in the past. Now I was having trouble thinking straight.

The teacher would give us pop quizzes on dosage calculations, and we weren't allowed to use calculators. Anything below 80 percent was a fail (because of the possibility of causing death). On one occasion there were six or seven of us writing a test in the nursing lounge. Initially, I looked at the ten questions on the sheet in front of me and thought, "I've got this." So why was my heart beating so fast? And was I . . . *sweating*? What I can only describe as a feeling of doom settled over me. Then my fight-or-flight instinct kicked in—or rather just the flight part. I jumped out of my seat and ran out of the room, knocking my desk over as I did so. I couldn't believe I was having my first heart attack at age twenty-one.

After calming me down, my teacher called my mom and Jordan, who came to pick me up. I felt embarrassed. We didn't talk about depression or anxiety in my family, at least not using those words. Even when I learned that what I had gone through was a panic attack—something 5 percent of the population will experience—it still felt like a moral rather than a physical failure. When the same sense of impending doom began to come on before clinicals, I got a script for anti-anxiety medication. But I had no one to talk to, neither counsellor nor friend, and was essentially self-diagnosing.

After that incident, I still had to take the dosage quizzes, but my teacher exempted me from being graded. In hindsight, it makes me angry that the school put such pressure on us. In the real world, a nurse estimating IV dosages isn't going to be scrawling calculations on a napkin; they'll be using a calculator (the last time I checked, these work even during a power outage). Then as now, high-alert medications require double sign-off, and yet the quizzes still call for manual calculations.

MY FIRST CODE BLUE happened while I was doing clinicals in med-surg. I was partnered as usual with a preceptor when we heard the Code Blue called. This usually means cardiac arrest. "Shit, that's *my* patient's room," I thought.

When nurses on *ER* or *Grey's Anatomy* rush in for a code it's always with a crash cart. But as a student you rush in with . . . nothing. This didn't dawn on me until I reached the doorway of the room, which was already filling up with staff. As I stood there, frozen on the spot, someone yelled, "Go get the crash cart!"

I ran (we're not supposed to, but we always do) to get the cart, which is a kind of one-stop-shop for any code: it's got PPE, high-alert meds, saline, scalpels, fluids, intubation and IV supplies, a defibrillator, a backboard for doing compressions, a giant magnet that can stop a pacemaker, and the big-bore needles required to prop open the collapsed veins of a patient whose heart has stopped.

Someone grabbed the backboard and put it under the patient, who had turned a terrible shade of grey. Up until that point, I'd only seen chest compressions done on TV. The real thing is nothing like what they show on the screen. It's way more violent and visceral. To get the necessary recoil, you need to press down at least one and a half to two inches, which often breaks the patient's ribs. This is what happened in this instance, and it was horrifyingly loud, like a big stick being snapped in half. Reviving someone through compressions can take as long as half an hour, so a lot of switching out is required since just two minutes of this work will make a healthy person drip with sweat. At some point one of the nurses asked me if I wanted to have a go. I declined as politely as I could, afraid I'd hurt the patient or wouldn't perform the compression efficiently enough. "I'm just here to observe," I said meekly.

The sordid details of chest compressions hadn't been taught in class. The same goes for coffee-grounds emesis, which I also saw for the first time that day. During this experience, the patient vomits up old, coagulated blood from the intestines, a sign of internal bleeding. The blood is dark brown and lumpy (hence "coffee grounds"), unlike frank (fresh) blood, which is bright red. If the patient aspirates this blood, they can die.

Five minutes later (though it felt like an eternity), the area looked like a crime scene. The bedding had been pulled off haphazardly, there was blood on the walls, and equipment was scattered everywhere. It was a ward room, so a curtain was the only barrier between this horror show and the other patients, who, like me, seemed terrified. They would have heard a lot of loud talk about death and resuscitation. The patient, who was quite elderly, eventually regained a pulse and was sent to ICU. I don't know if he ever came back, though.

After an incident, nurses are supposed to have hot and cold debriefs. (A "hot" debrief happens right after a triggering event, a "cold" one after everyone has had the chance to process what occurred.) In this case, neither happened. The whole thing was just shrugged off, as if they were saying, "This is healthcare, baby." And students generally get nothing, despite the fact that they probably need debriefing the most, given their inexperience. For me, the whole thing had been traumatizing.

When I was a newbie, it used to blow my mind that nurses ate lunch right after incidents that really upset me. This was before I got desensitized and learned to brush off the trauma—and eat my spaghetti and meat sauce feeling as if nothing disturbing had happened. I'd like to say here that although we shove the trauma down deep, it never really disappears, and this unhealthy behaviour is the reason many of us need therapy.

In nursing school, we were told to try to achieve "distance." But there was no acknowledgement of our real emotions, and no advice on how to reconcile returning home to our families after witnessing traumatic events. I never understood why we weren't given strategies to deal with the mental health element of being, or learning to be, a nurse. This lack of support meant that a lot of student nurses like me ended up struggling.

In second year, I was still being treated for panic attacks. When I was scheduled to do a mental health rotation, I idealistically imagined it might shed some light on my personal experiences. But in many ways, it had the opposite effect.

Mental health wards are nothing like what you see in TV shows or movies. My ward was pretty quiet most of the time. Occasionally a patient would raise their voice, but the scene bore no resemblance to *One Flew Over the Cuckoo's Nest*.

I remember talking to a patient who seemed fine until she pulled out a magazine and started "reading" it upside down. She told me that she had met all these different movie stars. In school they tell you not to feed a patient's delusion, but as a student and a learner I was curious to see where the story could go. So I started asking questions. The patient was West Indian, like me, so it didn't surprise me when she started using biblical references. But then it got weird. She cited a familiar bible passage about "changing in the twinkling of an eye" and declared, "I'm changing right now!" She looked completely serious. I had never dealt with anyone who was going through psychosis, and her detachment from reality creeped me out and made me sad.

I had another patient who heard voices. When I asked her what they were saying (this is a required component of harm assessments), she started talking about seeing a shadow and I got really freaked out. As I mentioned earlier, I had watched way too many horror movies. I actually wondered if the patient could see and hear things I couldn't! When I felt my Christian beliefs starting to seep in, I knew I had to put a lid on it, fast.

One day at the end of a shift, I found myself in the elevator with a schizophrenic man from the hospital's outpatient clinic. He asked me where I lived and I gave him a vague answer. Next he started saying he wanted to go home with me and "make babies." He actually followed me when we got off the elevator. Luckily, Jordan was waiting for me outside, so the situation didn't escalate any further, but I was terrified. In retrospect, I'm sure the man was harmless. But we had never been taught safety plans as part of our training or been told how to behave in that kind of situation.

What upset me far more than the behaviour of these patients was the way they were stigmatized by the staff who had been trained to understand them. Some of the nurses treated their patients as if they were irredeemably nuts, not ill.

Instead of shedding light on mental illness, my experience at that facility only left me more confused and fearful than I already was. In the end, a strike at the hospital meant my clinical ended early. Maybe things would have been different if I stayed the entire time, but I wonder if they might have actually gotten worse.

In the years since, my understanding of mental health has changed considerably. My brother has bipolar disorder, my husband and my sons have ADHD and autism, and many of my family members have suffered from depression and anxiety, me included. Despite the commonness of these conditions, there's still a lot of stigma, so I spend a lot of time advocating for government funding, paid sick days, and workplace benefits, and making mental health part of universal healthcare.

PROFESSIONAL DEVELOPMENT IS a built-in part of many jobs. Teachers take professional development courses. Doctors have to complete a certain number of Continuing Medical Education (CME) credits. In some jurisdictions, nurses do this too, but in many others they're more like real estate agents, pharmacists, or lawyers in that they're self-regulated, accountable not to an exterior governing body but to our professional college (in the case of me and Sara, the College of Nurses of Ontario). The college ensures its members keep their educational standards up to date by doing random audits. We might be asked what independent research we've done, what non-mandatory courses we've taken, or how we've reflected on our practice.

One nurse who was in her sixties got audited by the College and was asked to write a paper that reflected her practice. She found this super stressful, especially when her paper got rejected. At the time she was at most a couple of years away from retirement. Auditing a nurse at that stage of her career made no sense to me, especially since none of the younger nurses I know (nor I) have been asked to do this (knock on wood!). Nursing's poor accountability structure affects us in other ways too. For example, part of my job as a nurse leader is to educate nurses on the latest evidence-based practices and technologies. They often resist this. And who can blame them? Other than the remote threat of an audit, there's not much motivation for learning this stuff. And they're given no dedicated time for this kind of learning.

So if I said, "Hey, Susie, we have an in-service here on pumps. Do you have ten minutes for me to show you how?" more often than not the reply was, "I haven't had lunch, I haven't had a sip of water, I haven't peed, and one of my seven patient needs to get prepped for diagnostic imaging while I deal with two new admissions" (which is basically a polite way of saying, "Fuck off"). There were some nurses who came to me at the end of their shift and offered to stay an extra ten minutes to learn about the pump (or whatever the thing in question was), even though they most likely wouldn't get paid for the time.

Nursing school still uses caring theories to promote the outdated idea that nurses are an angelic force and that like priests, we're called to our vocation—essentially, that we're martyrs. This is toxic and puts us in a bad place politically and socially. Nurses are the largest workforce in healthcare, but have the smallest say in how healthcare is run. We're expected not to complain, to be thankful we have jobs and the honour of looking after people. It should be possible to feel privileged to work in your chosen field yet also refuse to be somebody's doormat or punching bag.

The fact that the job is still predominantly female feeds into the whole "caring" narrative, and it's also reflected in the very word *nursing*, which has heavy maternal connotations. Over four years, that kind of language starts to feel demeaning. We're seen as "ladies of the lamp," wielders of knowledge and art (with maybe a sprinkling of science). A lot of women go into nursing because they feel disempowered, but when they get there they find themselves at the bottom of a strict hierarchical ladder, handmaidens to physicians at the top.

A lot of nurses I know have swallowed that Kool-Aid. They get offended when we call nursing a job instead of a calling. They don't see that these martyrish attitudes are detrimental to the profession, that they stop us from being seen as the experts in our field that we are and and that they limit our ability to vocalize concerns and frustrations. Would an angel-martyr ask for better wages and sick days, or complain about violence or verbal abuse in the workplace?

Addressing inequities in the profession and in healthcare itself—the fact that major parts of society don't receive the care to which they're entitled—needs to start at ground zero: in nursing school. Instead of asking nursing students to regurgitate airy-fairy caring theories drummed up by (predominantly) white women, why aren't we encouraging them to ask open-ended questions like how to incorporate the social determinants of health into caring, or to advocate for better outcomes for patients (and nurses themselves)?

NURSE WITH GRIT

Cori Bush (b. 1976)

In 2021, Cori Bush—registered nurse, single mother, Black Lives Matter activist, and ordained pastor—ended a half-century political dynasty when she beat Rep. William Lacy Clay to become the Democratic US representative for Missouri's First Congressional District. Bush knew from personal and professional experience the ways racism in health-care could affect people and even threaten their lives. In May 2021, she testified to the House Oversight and Reform Committee that she had gone into pre-term labour after her doctor ignored her complaints of severe pain. Bush, who at the time was living out of her car, saw the treatment she had received as typical of what Black women in the US regularly face during pregnancy and childbirth. Shortly after her testimony, she summed it up in a Tweet: "Every day, Black birthing people and our babies die because our doctors don't believe our pain. My children almost became a statistic. I almost became a statistic [...] Hear us. Believe us. Because for so long, nobody has."

If we have a chance to change such statistics it will be because nurses like Cori Bush are not being afraid to take on positions of real power.

Sara

I've been a patient far fewer times than Amie (which, to be clear, is a contest I'm happy to lose!). But though my experiences have been limited to the births of my children, both were eye-opening in different ways, good and bad, professionally and personally.

I had my first child at the maternity ward of a Toronto hospital where I previously worked in postpartum and the NICU. This alone would have made it a strange experience, like going for dinner at the restaurant where you work as a server in the daytime. You want to relax, but you can't help noticing all the stuff that regular customers don't: the bus pans, the coffee station, the anxious kitchen staff—or in my case, the IV pump settings, the fetal heart monitor, even how often nurses chart on the computer. I especially took notice of how (or if) they explained things to me.

It was 6 a.m. when my water broke. I was a couple of days over 37 weeks, so a bit before my official due date.

I wasn't having any contractions, which meant I would have to be induced. Knowing how slow a first labour typically is, I took a taxi to the hospital.

(The second time, my husband, Kevin, drove me to the hospital, but the birth was still as protracted as the first, about twelve hours long. As far as I know, I'm pretty much the only person whose second labour wasn't any faster than the first! For both, I was able to get an epidural and deliver "naturally," a.k.a. vaginally.)

I worked mostly on the postpartum floor, so while my surroundings were familiar, the staff who greeted me weren't. In fact, I didn't know anyone. I never announced that I was a nurse or that I had worked there previously, but I knew my profession was written on my chart. At the time, I was working as a clinical nurse specialist at another hospital. The nurse assigned to me definitely knew this, because we talked about what I did and didn't want for the birth. I'm certain this awareness influenced what happened when my baby's heart rate suddenly, and alarmingly, dropped.

At this point I was in active labour and hooked up to all the various monitors. After glancing at these, the nurse—who was middle-aged and had a distinct air of authority—reached down to touch my belly. It was hard as a rock. The oxytocin I'd been getting via IV to speed up my labour had worked too well: my body was now over-contracting. We both knew how dangerous this was: if the uterus stays contracted too long, it can cut off blood flow to the baby, potentially causing brain damage. If things didn't improve fast, I'd be headed for a crash C-section in the OR.

The nurse gave me a worried look before turning me on my side. The machine monitoring the baby's heart rate was now making a shrill sound that I knew would be picked up on the screens at the nurses' station and bring members of the healthcare team running in preparation for possible resuscitation or surgery.

Almost as soon as I was able to form this thought, a crowd started gathering in the room. A bad sign. I heard someone whisper, "She used to work here. *Nothing* goes wrong!"

Because the monitors were behind me, I wasn't actually aware that my baby's heart rate had dropped. But Kevin, who was standing off to the side, could see it clearly. He looked shell-shocked and on the brink of tears.

I was instructed to flip side to side to get the baby's heart rate up, which I did diligently. I remember the nurse said she'd never seen anyone with an epidural move so quickly (I was technically frozen from the waist down).

But although I appeared calm, inside I was panicking. I'd recently written the protocol for the hospital where I worked on what to do in an obstetrical emergency, and I considered the irony that this same code might be called on me!

Eventually, people started to trickle out of the room (a good sign) as the emergency passed. Although I was super thankful to the team for their quick actions, their communication skills left something to be desired. They hadn't talked that much to me during the incident, neither when things were going badly nor when they got better. This is when being a nurse at the receiving end of treatment can be a mixed bag. A "regular" patient would never have been treated like my husband and I were treated. There seemed to be an assumption that because I was a nurse, I didn't need support or hand-holding. But being on the other side of the nurse-patient equation can be really disorienting, especially when the occasion is your first birth. Having a calm, empathetic voice to ground you and keep you informed of what's going on is always helpful.

For Kevin, on the other hand, the entire experience was traumatizing. Because no one explained to him that things had gotten back on track, he remained under the impression that he was witnessing an emergency of the highest order. (In the end it was me who reassured him that we were out of danger.) Kevin is a numbers guy, so he coped by focusing on the fetal heart monitor, which gave him concrete, reliable information and a clear plan of action: if the heart rate dipped below a certain level, he knew his job was to go get a nurse.

As for me, I felt that no one was seeing me as a person who hadn't experienced this momentous life event before. They saw me instead as a liability and a number—specifically, the number representing my baby's heartbeat. Maybe they assumed I *did* know his heart rate had gone down, and that I knew what my role was and how I should behave. But even if the assumption was that I did know, that's no excuse for not keeping me in the loop, for treating me as a patient, not a nurse. I've always believed it's important to debrief a patient after they experience a stressful situation and enable them to access the information in their health records (in healthcare we're always worried that when a patient asks for their chart it's because they want to sue the hospital).

As Amie said, deciding whether to disclose that you're a nurse can feel like a major quandary when you're hospitalized or receiving care. During that birth, I think disclosure ultimately worked against me. In other situations, however, self-disclosing can be an advantage. When nurses know they're treating another nurse, they're likely to do everything by the book and not cut any corners. One of the downsides to self-disclosing is that you might be seen as high maintenance, especially if you start suggesting "better" ways to do things.

My nursing knowledge and expertise definitely helped me in postpartum situations, such as when my first child developed jaundice shortly after birth and had to be readmitted overnight for phototherapy. Jaundice is quite common in East Asian babies. I had it, so I was half-expecting it in my own kids. The condition has three levels of severity. The first level of jaundice resolves by itself. The second level usually gets better with phototherapy, which involves "bathing" the baby in a special light for up to 24 hours in an isolette (a.k.a. an incubator). The third and most severe level can require blood transfusions. Without transfusions, elevated levels of bilirubin in the baby's bloodstream can cause brain damage, hearing loss, and vision problems.

My son was in the middle category and would therefore need phototherapy. I helped set up his isolette and put on the little goggles and foam eye covers that would protect his newborn eyes from harmful rays. He looked like a cute space creature on one of those old-fashioned tanning beds. The process might have caused anxiety in other new parents, but I was calm, knowing from experience that everything was going to be just fine.

It was a different story when it came to nursing my son. I had helped countless mothers establish breastfeeding in my work in mother-baby care and as a lactation consultant. Now I needed outside help as well. My milk was key to resolving my son's jaundice, but it wasn't coming in fast enough. The nurse had to hand-express my breast quite hard just to get a few drops of milk out. At one point a breast pump was suggested, but I didn't end up needing one.

AS FOR THE actual birth, my training in labour and delivery helped me . . . but only to a point. When it comes to the pain of the birthing process, your perspective *really* shifts when the tables are turned.

As a prenatal educator, I had preached the benefits of natural childbirth to parents and provided mothers with pain-reduction strategies. Then I felt the pain myself firsthand, and all bets were off. When I arrived at the hospital, I was only six centimetres dilated, nowhere near ready to push. The staff got me into a room and left me there for 45 minutes.

By the time they came back, I had tossed all those well-meaning pain-reduction strategies out the window, not to mention my birthing plan, and was essentially begging for an epidural.

The anaesthesiologist arrived soon afterwards, but before inserting the long needle into my spine that would give me relief, he launched into the long legal spiel that was required of him. He had a resident with him, so he went into what seemed like more detail than usual explaining the procedure, including its risks, which of course I knew. He explained how my back worked, noting that I had mild scoliosis. (No one ever followed up with me on this bedside diagnosis. It also wasn't mentioned when I got an epidural for my second child.) All the while I was in agony. The final requirement was signing the waiver form, which had to be done between contractions (it isn't easy to hold a pen, let alone sign your name, when one of those massive waves passes through you). When my child's heartbeat had slowed down, I wanted more information; now I wanted less, and for the anaesthesiologist to get on with the show.

If an epidural isn't inserted in the right spot, there's a chance you'll get little to no pain relief, so you have to stay very still when receiving it. I nailed that part. Once the anaesthesia started flowing, I felt instantly better. It amazed me that pain so intense and all-encompassing could just disappear. All power to those women who opt for natural birth—I didn't turn out to be one of them, and I'm fine with that. In the moment, I realized I had nothing to prove to anyone, especially myself.

When you're a nurse coping with a medical issue, a little knowledge can go a long way, as was the case with my son's jaundice. On the other hand, too much knowledge can create anxiety, as anyone who's ever googled a medical condition knows. Before I had my second child, I regularly reviewed cases where things had gone horribly wrong during pregnancy and labour, like injuries caused during forceps or vacuum deliveries, or an amniotic fluid embolism, a rare condition that can be fatal for the mother either during or after birth. I worried that I'd give birth prematurely and that my baby, like many preemies, would have chronic respiratory problems or physical and mental disabilities. I worried about the possibility of a C-section, having cared for a patient whose incision became so infected we had to bring in a plastic surgeon and put a container of charcoal in the room to absorb the smell.

It took a lot of effort not to go to these dark places during my pregnancy, no matter how low the statistical probabilities. Thankfully, for me as for most women, my fears were unfounded, and my two kids were born normal and healthy.

AS AMIE POINTED out earlier, patients who are doctors, lawyers, and teachers tend to raise red flags with nurses (lawyers being the most terrifying because they can sue you free of charge if they're not happy with your care). One of the most difficult patients I ever had was a lawyer in her fifties who had gotten pregnant via a donor egg and sperm. Lawyers, in my experience, feel anxious when they're in a situation they can't control, and this woman was the embodiment of this theory. She had a type-A personality and was incredibly high strung. Everything had to be done a certain way and delivered *now*. She arrived with a four-page-long birth plan and very detailed instructions for breastfeeding and baby care. If we suggested an alternative way of doing something—whether it was feeding, swaddling, or bathing the baby—she simply wasn't interested, no matter how strong the scientific evidence backing it up.

I had another patient who refused everything. No blood pressure checks, even though she had high blood pressure. No blood-sugar checks on the baby, even though she had gestational diabetes, which put her baby at risk of low blood sugar. Her doctor was aware of all of this and told me to just abide by her wishes. Since he had medically signed off on her decisions, there wasn't much I could do to help her. Very frustrating!

You'll notice nurses aren't on our list of difficult-to-treat professionals (although there are definitely a few who are a handful). That's because, for the most part, nurses rarely demand special treatment like a private room (unlike a lot of doctors). My own experiences treating nurses—the ones I *knew* were nurses, that is—have almost always been positive, the exception being labour and delivery nurses like me. When you're helping a woman who specializes in labour and delivery with her own labour and delivery, there's pressure to do everything perfectly in order to avoid criticism. But some of these fears may be just in my head. I think most nurses would agree with me that, overall, we make excellent patients!

Nurse Papa

When we bathe these children, we are gentle and kind. There is no hurry or haste. We may softly sing songs that we know they liked and once sang along with us. If they still have the hair on their heads, we brush it until it appears as they once preferred it to be. As we clean their limbs, torso, and face, we sometimes laugh or smile as we remember funny things they said or did. We talk to these kids too—like we would have when they were still alive—and we are content when they do not reply as they once might have. "I'm going to clean your face now, sweetie," I remember saying once to a child who could not possibly answer back.

—DAVID METZGER, *Nurse Papa*

As an RN in pediatric oncology at UCSF Children's Hospital in San Francisco, David Metzger long ago accepted death as a sad but unavoidable part of his work. In the passage above from his memoir, *Nurse Papa*, he describes what it's like to bathe the body of a deceased child. It's an intimate ritual, but one that not every parent is comfortable doing. But for those who decide to take it on, it can be powerfully symbolic. A parent may not have had the power to rid their child of disease in life, but in death they can cleanse their child's pain-free body in a controlled, loving way.

David recalls seeing a mother howling in agony and fresh grief, throwing her body over that of her deceased teenage daughter. Once she began the process of washing her daughter's body, however, her demeanor changed completely. She became a mom again. Calm and focused, she asked staff for some warm water, then adjusted the temperature several times until it was just right. She washed and styled her daughter's hair and gave her a manicure. When she was done, nurses took her daughter's body down to the morgue.

BEING A DAD to two young kids and working in pediatric oncology means that David is a caregiver both at work and at home. Inhabiting these dual roles can also create moments of cognitive dissonance. For instance, he might wash a dead child's body at work, then come home and give his own children a riotous, sudsy bath. Likewise, the motion of picking up his sleeping kids and putting them to bed can recall the act of placing a child's body on a tray in the morgue. In both cases, the child will bear a serene expression, but only one will wake up. For David, what unites these acts is a sense of intimacy and privilege.

Caring for kids with cancer takes a special kind of person. (David's patients range from infants to people in their twenties who developed cancer when they were younger and relapsed.) It's one thing to work in long-term care, or even with adults with cancer. There's sadness there, but it's different from the sadness attached to a terminally ill child. Most of us can't think of anything worse than our child dying before we do.

Cancer, and its treatment, can strain what we understand about the relationship between mind and body. David has seen the transformation countless times. A patient arrives newly diagnosed, still looking like a typical kid. After a year of treatment, they're unrecognizable. Dark, shiny hair has been reduced to pale, patchy tufts. Skin that was resilient and flush is now papery and translucent. Plump lips have shrivelled and become chapped. Healthy limbs have slowly grown weak from inactivity.

And yet these children, even with their bald heads and skinny bodies, have struck David time and again with their beauty and incredible strength of spirit. Most will still smile and giggle, talk about their hopes and dreams. The body might be sick, but the spirit stays strong.

Sometimes their losses turn into gains. An example was when David watched a teen called Alex go through the long, painful process of salvaging his cancer-ridden leg with surgically implanted titanium rods. (The decision of whether or not to save a limb is strongly influenced by the institution or the surgeon treating the child, as well as the type and stage of cancer; some physicians support preservation, others not so much.) Alex retained the leg, but he was miserable. A few years later, David encountered Alex again during a visit to the hospital. His leg had been amputated, and he told David that he was now playing soccer with his new prosthetic limb. He and his mother both seemed so much happier. This raises the question: What, ultimately, makes us who we are? For Alex, was part of it the process of realizing he should amputate his leg?

Because so many of his patients die, David can't always see his role as that of healer. With a patient who will likely die from cancer, the question David asks himself becomes, What kind of person am I going to be for that child during the precious time they have left?

He admits he has moments of magical thinking. When you get to know a person well, as David does with so many of his patients, there's a tendency to imagine they will always be there, even when their condition is so severe they essentially have no chance of survival. On more than one occasion he's looked at the face of a child who has passed away expecting them to open their eyes.

And yet when he talks about his work it's mostly in happy, joyful terms. He considers the natural curiosity he's had about people ever since he was a child growing up in Orange County, California, (he is now in his forties) to be an occupational advantage. "I get to talk all day to people, have conversations about things that are important, or stupid. It's so much fun." He loves helping his patients to be their authentic selves, loves to become interested in whatever they're interested in, to laugh about the same things. It's easy to imagine these interactions when you hear his warm, reassuring voice and see his easy smile.

And there really are laughs. Like the time that, while checking on a young boy named Tony, he reached down to rub Tony's foot to comfort him, only to realize that the "foot" was in fact the toe of Tony's grandma, who'd been asleep next to him and was now awake, chuckling.

Or the time David was helping a young man named Ben prepare for a bone marrow transplant. The therapy necessary for this procedure is so powerful it can kill a patient. So when alerts on all the monitors Ben was hooked up to started to go off, David ran into the room, fully expecting to find him unresponsive. When he arrived, he found Ben happily sitting in bed watching a basketball game. Relieved, David left, but the alerts went off again a few minutes later. That's when the penny dropped: every time the point guard on his favourite team made a shot, Ben—totally wrapped up in the game—was holding his breath!

One of the funniest lines David ever heard in his life came from the mother of Chloe, a teenage girl who was dying. David had come into

Chloe's room to help Danielle, who was her nurse that day. Danielle was in the process of adjusting Chloe's medication pump to give her an extra dose of morphine when Chloe's mom said to David, "I see you have a woody, and poo on your shirt too." Shocked by the inappropriate comment, Danielle whipped her head towards David, but she didn't see what she had visualized. Instead, she realized what Chloe's mother was referring to: two patches on David' scrubs, one of Winnie-the-Pooh holding a honey pot and another of Woody from *Toy Story*. Chloe's mom had nothing to laugh about, but in the moment she chose to break the tension with a perfectly timed joke.

BEFORE HE EVER considered nursing as a career, David trained as a painter and sculptor. In art school, he learned how to look at things deeply. To ask questions like: What am I trying to portray emotionally? What's my purpose? How is the light hitting that object? What if I angled things another way?

He applies the same kind of thinking when he encounters a new patient. He uses his eyes to assess the child and to read the room's emotional temperature. Then he'll ask himself a series of questions: Is the patient's skin colour good or bad? How do they want me to engage with them? How are mom and dad doing? How can I place myself in this canvas therapeutically?

Children with cancer are often in hospital for many months at a time. Collectively, these stays can add up to years. Some parents view this time as one of stasis. But while a child who's spent most of their life in an institution certainly isn't going to receive the same stimuli as other kids, David points out that they're still growing, making mistakes, maturing, and acquiring wisdom. A life doesn't need to be long to be meaningful. David recalls one parent gushing about how proud she was of her son's accomplishments. He had excelled in school, but she wasn't talking about academics. She was referring to his bravery in facing his disease, to the fact that he'd never once complained.

He mentions Madeleine, a patient with trisomy 21 (Down's syndrome) and leukemia who was in hospital for a long time, but who was extremely high functioning. Madeleine's mom credited this to one-on-one learning in a sheltered environment with lots of interpersonal communication.

Over the fifteen years he's been in oncology, David has become used to talking about uncomfortable subjects. When he was a less experienced nurse, though, David often found it awkward to observe the pain of others. A child or a parent would be crying in front of him and he had no idea what to do or say. But in time, he came to realize that the awkwardness was his, not theirs. What he needed to do was encounter the moment, tell the person he hurt for them, that they were not alone in their pain.

He also learned that kids' pain can be as much existential as physical. When he sees that this is the case, he focuses on being a calming presence. He will kneel next to his patients to get to their eye level. As with many of his patient interactions, this isn't something he was trained to do. Rather, it's something he remembers his father doing when he delivered the news that David's grandfather had died. What David took away from that exchange wasn't shock or sadness, but the feeling of safety he got from his father's closeness. It's a feeling he tries to convey to his patients, who are so often frightened and bewildered.

The first sick child he ever encountered as a nursing student was a two-year-old girl whose entire body was covered in painful red lesions, symptoms of a (curable) auto-immune disease called Stevens-Johnson syndrome. The girl was all alone and shrieking at the top of her lungs, gripping the edge of her hospital crib. The nurse mentoring him that day gave David an assignment: stay by her side and calm her down.

Easier said than done. With no idea how to accomplish his task, David turned to instinct, as he would many times throughout his career. He gathered the girl into his arms and sang to her. The effect was immediate and miraculous. Looking directly into his eyes, her nose and eyes a river of snot and tears, the girl stopped crying. If he stopped singing she'd start again, so he kept it up until she finally fell asleep on his shoulder, exhausted. The girl's problem wasn't pain but fear. In the end, all she needed was a reassuring hug and a silly made-up song.

ADOLESCENCE IS TOUGH at the best of times, let alone when you have cancer, so it's understandable that some male patients feel more comfortable opening up to David about their personal problems than to a female nurse. There was Mike, who was dealing with the dual challenges of a brain tumour and recently being dumped by his girlfriend. On top of this, Mike had decided to bank his sperm prior to getting chemo, but he had been unable to masturbate into a cup. "It's way too much pressure," he told David. David assured him that his issue wasn't uncommon and that if the tables were turned he would surely have the same problem.

David has always tried hard to put himself in the shoes of the kids he treats, as well as their parents' shoes, to imagine what it's like to feel their pain. Before he was a parent, he did his job with the heart of the father he hoped to be.

Then six years in, he became a father himself.

Being a dad completely changed David's understanding of his patients. It also seemed to change their understanding of him. "I wear that parenthood thing on my forehead. I'll start talking about my kids in a way that lets parents know that I get what they're going through. After that, it's amazing how quickly people let down their guard and unload."

Years ago, David adopted from one of his favourite doctors the habit of wearing colourful wristbands around the neck of his stethoscope. This positive visual display—each band bears the name of a patient and a declaration of hope—always seems to put new parents and patients at ease.

David began to imagine himself as a whole new entity called "Nurse Papa," a guise that embodies the very real and sometimes intense cross-connection between his experience as a children's nurse and a dad to his own kids (*Nurse Papa* is the title of his book and the name of the popular podcast he hosts). He might apply the redirection techniques he uses on his own kids to calm an agitated patient or use his nursing experience to reassure his kids when they're afraid or in pain. The nature of his job means David's experiences with children have been, in many ways, the reverse of most people's. Before he had kids himself, he was far more familiar with how sick children looked and acted than healthy ones.

Some of lessons he tries to carry over from work into parenting are living in the moment, accepting that bad things happen, and knowing that we can learn from them. Although he doesn't consider himself a parenting expert, David tends not to sweat the small stuff. He takes what he calls a "free-range" approach to parenting. This means allowing his kids to sustain the odd bruise or scrape, and to get into iffy situations just so they can learn to find their way out of them. In his communications with his kids, he is straightforward and open. His only real expectation is that they try to be good people. And like any parent, sometimes he thinks he's doing a great job only to have his confidence shaken when he loses his temper, or when his kids say something hurtful that gets to him more than it should.

FOR THE PARENTS of a child with cancer, mourning can begin at the moment of diagnosis. From then on, the losses pile up. No first day of school. No hair to tie into a ponytail. No sending them off to prom. Anger is a common reaction, and on the odd occasion when David finds himself at the receiving end of it, he doesn't take it personally. He aims to forge positive relationships with parents, even when they're difficult or disruptive. "I always try to meet them where they are. What they want is to be heard rather than to have something fixed, to acknowledge that what's happening is fucked up." Sometimes all it takes to break through is to ask how their day went and to nod sympathetically when they give the inevitable answer: "Horrible."

The untold stress of cancer treatment means that even when the child survives, the parents' marriage sometimes doesn't. Minor differences of opinion can get wildly magnified. David once heard a couple, whose daughter had a rare form of cancer called neuroblastoma, fighting in the room where she slept. The father kept yelling at the top of his lungs, "There is no fucking heaven!" The parents of another patient vowed that they would die by suicide if their son passed away. Fortunately he survived, but David never doubted the parents' determination to kill themselves.

Because nurses are an integral part of a child's support system while they are treated, carriers of their emotional burdens and witnesses to their journey, many parents over time come to see them as part of the family. David finds this touching but also sad. He knows many parents will mourn his loss as well after their child is gone.

A child's reaction to a sibling's illness will be quite different from that of their parents. On the day a little girl named Lucia died, her parents and extended family sat gathered around her body, speaking in hushed tones. Wearing her favourite red flowered dress, brown curls framing her cute, chubby face, Lucia looked as beatific as she had in life.

Absent from this group was Lucia's younger sister, Veronica, whom David had come to recognize over the year he treated Lucia. She was outside in the hallway, seemingly playing happily with an inflatable ball she kept bouncing off the walls. David could even hear her singing.

As he walked past her on his way to attend to a patient, he listened in. The tune, which she was repeating over and over, was a familiar nursery rhyme, but the words had changed to "My sister is an angel. My sister is an angel. My sister is an angel." Sensing David's attention, the little girl stopped playing and looked at him, her expression somewhere between trust and indifference. Then she turned away and resumed her singing and ball-bouncing.

Although that look confused him at the time, David would come to recognize it later in his own children. It was the look of a child who has had a profound experience for which they have not yet found words. For his part, David found himself deeply moved by the contrast between the beauty of Veronica's song and the sadness of the event that had precipitated it—Lucia's death.

WHEN CANCER IS terminal, the march towards death is often sadly predictable, a gradual chipping away at personality and autonomy. Sometimes the slowness of the journey can be a kind of gift, a time for the patient to be with the people they love and to choose how they want the rest of their life to play out. Because this phase is so intense, David and his colleagues form profound relationships much more quickly than would normally be the case.

Despite his obvious thoughtfulness, David, who grew up Jewish but isn't religious, says he doesn't adhere to any specific philosophy about life and death. And yet there's a distinct spiritual tinge to the way he talks about his work and life; about how he's managed to find beauty in the process of transformation that happens with death; about how when it comes to that process, nursing can have such a consequential effect on someone's experience.

Adults who are dying will often talk in metaphorical language about packing their bags and taking a trip. Kids who are dying also say things that are fanciful and seemingly unconstrained by reality. Once, a little girl said something to David about going to a beach and flying away. Simple and sweet as the words were, he immediately knew she wasn't talking about a future parasailing vacation; she was talking about her own imminent death.

Most actively dying patients, including children, end up on powerful pain medication cocktails that leave them lethargic or barely conscious. In David's experience, some of the most sublime moments happen in the slender margin between life and death, when a child is still conscious, perhaps holding a parent's hand and talking, but not in pain or struggling. How a child approaches the end of their life depends, like so many things, on their developmental age. Teens have more agency to run the show. Little kids, on the other hand, tend to want to please their parents, sometimes to the extent of hanging on to life to protect the people they love and depend on the most.

The first time David witnessed this, he was a young nurse caring for a dying teenager named Theo. As Theo lay sleeping, his anxious father hovered around him. After a while, the experienced nurse David was working with asked the father: "Have you told him it's all right to go? That you'll be okay when he does?"

David was shocked by the bluntness of the question. But it turned out to be exactly what that father needed to hear. Just as he would have once given Theo permission to go to the corner store, he now needed to give him permission to leave his mortal coil. For David, it was a lesson about the importance of saying difficult but necessary things.

Kids are often unable to fully engage with their own complex feelings about their illness. David met Jason when he was admitted to the hospital for a liver transplant. During surgery prep, however, a massive tumour was discovered inside Jason's abdomen, making him ineligible for the procedure.

After this news, Jason basically shut down. He withdrew from the world and no longer communicated in a functional way. Instead of talking to David or the other staff, he whispered requests to his dad, an unconventional person who often said strange things. (In David's eyes, this made him in many ways the perfect person to deal with the painful and scary situation his son was facing.) At the time, David's wife was pregnant with their second child, and he often reflected on the hope he felt about bringing another child into a world that Jason, due to his physical and emotional pain, could no longer fully engage with.

Because even modest exertion left him exhausted, Jason had refused to be bathed for many days (in fairness, having a shower must have felt entirely trivial to him at that point). David, knowing that bathing is as much about comfort as it is about infection control, kept gently coaxing the teen until he finally agreed.

David soon found himself in an intimate, awkward dance with a fully naked Jason. As they stood face to face, Jason's bony arms draped limply over David's shoulders, two other nurses slowly and carefully washed the teen's body. Afterwards, David gently lowered a relaxed, sweet-smelling Jason into his freshly made bed. As the boy lay back, his arms behind his head, it struck David that Jason looked more like a sunbather relaxing on a beach than a dying boy in a hospital bed.

That afternoon, after Jason's parents left for the day, David had a rare moment alone with the teen in his room. Late-summer sun was filtering through the windows, creating a womb-like atmosphere as

David occupied himself charting. He could hear Jason's quiet breathing and assumed he was sleeping. But then David looked up and, for what felt like the first time, found Jason meeting his gaze directly. The connection felt startling, meaningful.

"David?"

He held his breath. Jason had never used his name before.

"Do you have any pets?"

David smiled. "Yeah, we have a cat, but she doesn't get much attention these days because of our new baby," he replied.

"We had three cats, but we had to put one down because she was old and wouldn't eat," Jason said.

"I'm sorry you lost your cat. That's sad."

"It is. But if you love cats, you have to be okay with it."

The sentiment behind these words was profound and undeniable. We're all going to die, but if you love life, you have to be okay with that. More profound still was the fact that Jason couldn't talk about himself this way, but he could channel his emotions through the story of a dead pet. It sounded like a line out of a movie. David imagined the director calling, "Cut!"

Jason died two weeks later. Shortly after, David started writing *Nurse Papa*.

ACCORDING TO RESEARCH, the trauma nurses experience on the job isn't that different from what soldiers experience during war. The brain wants to shut itself off and disengage emotionally, to say, "Okay, I'll do my job, but at a remove."

For six years David had managed to find a good work/life balance. He focused on staying healthy by exercising regularly. If he felt he needed to work something out but wasn't quite sure what it was, he talked to his colleagues or grabbed his paddleboard and headed for San Francisco Bay.

But when Jason died, these usual outlets no longer seemed to work. The joy and sense of purpose David used to be able to access appeared to be slipping away.

So he turned to another latent skill, writing, and found the process to be both cathartic and therapeutic. He finished his book and started a podcast about his experience as a parent and a nurse to sick children. Telling stories and having conversations "thawed that freezer inside me. I saw it on people's faces. Their reactions made me remember what it was like to feel those intense human emotions for the first time, and to be moved and changed by them once they were over."

Nurses are full of stories, and David thinks that even those who aren't naturally gifted with a pen or a keyboard can benefit from telling them. "You're working out a puzzle when you're writing, and though I didn't realize it at the time, writing put wind into my sails. Going so deep added layers of richness to my life. I don't think I am any more fearful than other people, but the act of writing about these sick kids and admitting some hard truths about my limitations as a dad required a lot of courage. It was hard. Once I did it though, in a book that so many people read, I found out that many nurses and parents could relate to the same emotional challenges. That feeling of togetherness continues to amaze me, and I am grateful for it."

Amie

Ever since I became a nurse, I feel like a cloud is hanging over my head when I'm out and about, like some random medical event or accident is going to happen, forcing me to jump in and save the day. The feeling is especially strong when I'm with my husband, Jordan, probably because when something does happen he always pushes me to get involved, saying it's my ethical responsibility (although when I hear him bragging that I'm his wife, I get the distinct impression that there's some personal pride involved too).

To be clear, I *do* feel the ethical pull to help. But I also feel a very human fear. Fear of being attacked or hurt myself, and of the risks of treating people outside healthcare walls. Inside those walls we have resources, teams, and supplies to fall back on for support. But in a "Good Samaritan" situation, you must rely on your judgment, your skills, and your ability to keep calm while waiting for the ambulance to arrive.

The thing is, these incidents happen. I've attended to people who collapsed at funerals and malls and parks and airports and neighbours' homes. For a while, these incidents were happening so frequently that I started carrying medical supplies with me. In my car I have gloves, wound-cleaning supplies, a suture kit, a CPR kit, and—compliments of the expired medicine storage room at my hospital—18- and 20-gauge IV needles and a saline lock. (As with many foods, the expiry date on medical supplies is a suggestion or recommendation—not to mention a way for medical-supply companies to make more money. Needles, for instance, basically never expire.)

While there are Good Samaritan laws in place to protect people who offer aid from liability, it's always best if possible to obtain consent before treating somebody. If I'm in a restaurant and the person next to me starts choking (it has happened), I will intervene if they signal for help or lose consciousness. If they are truly choking, they'll be unable to cough. It's always best if the person ejects the obstruction themselves. If you intervene while they're coughing, you risk lodging the item even deeper into their windpipe.

When they're not on the job, every nurse needs to decide for themselves how far they will go to assist a stranger. I've never turned away when someone needed help, but I usually feel some reluctance to get drawn into a stranger's drama (I also hate being the centre of attention). I always hope a doctor will step up before I do, but in my experience so far—except for one time when I was on a plane—it's always me who steps up.

I'm not the only one who has these fears. A lot of people are hesitant to treat a stranger. Administering mouth-to-mouth—the whole two breaths, thirty compressions, two breaths—is particularly scary. Recognizing this problem, in 2020 the Heart and Stroke Foundation started a new campaign: if you encounter someone who is having a cardiac arrest and requires resuscitation, at least do the compressions. With cardiac arrest, it's not about the respiratory system; it's about restarting the heart, and even a hundred compressions may help the individual survive.

A person who is actively bleeding can die in as little as five minutes. The US-based Stop the Bleed initiative was created in response to the 2012 Sandy Hook Elementary School shooting. It also addresses the general phenomenon of people's wariness about performing CPR on collision or accident victims. The 90-minute course, now available in Canada, teaches participants basic nursing skills like stopping blood loss, packing a wound, and using a tourniquet.

As I've gotten older and more experienced, I've also become less apprehensive about nursing on the fly. When I find I'm hesitating, I ask myself: If I were in this situation, would I want someone to help me? The answer is invariably *yes*.

I also think about my uncle, who was killed while riding his motor-cycle when he was T-boned as he drove legally through a four-way stop. When I spoke to the coroner, I was told that people at the scene of the accident had stopped and tried to help him, which was a huge source of comfort to me and my family.

The choice to intervene isn't always clear cut. Someone who is choking or passing out, or has been in a roadside accident in front of you, is one thing. But let's say you're walking down the beach and you pass someone who has a strange growth on their back. Do you stop and say something?

In October 2021, a twenty-two-year-old nursing assistant named Nadia Popovici did just that. Popovici was at a Vancouver Canucks game in Seattle when she spotted a two-centimetre mole on the neck of Brian Hamilton, the team's assistant equipment manager. When the game ended, she directed Hamilton's attention to a typed message on her cell phone: "The mole on the back of your neck is possibly cancerous. Please go see a doctor!" The words *mole*, *cancer*, and *doctor* were in red.

Although she later admitted that she worried the interaction was inappropriate, Popovici was vindicated when Hamilton got tested and discovered that the mole was type 2 malignant melanoma. Popovici's message literally saved Hamilton's life. Much was made of this feel-good story in the press after Hamilton tracked Popovici down via social media to thank her. At a subsequent game, the two hockey teams presented her with a $10,000 cheque for her medical school expenses.

There is nothing ambiguous about that story. But it could just as easily happen that you raise a flag and cause someone weeks of stress, only to learn that test results are negative. Obesity puts people at high risk for many conditions. Should nurses stop them on the street and tell them their odds for diabetes or heart disease? The choice between minding my own business and being punched in the face is, for me anyway, an easy one!

When it comes to medical topics, very little fazes us nurses (though I personally draw the line at pediatric surgery—and my tolerance went down further after I had children). We'll talk about the grossest stuff, even over a meal. Our favourite TV shows, websites, and YouTube channels run the gamut between gross and outright dark: *Dr. Pimple Popper*, *Trauma: Life in the ER*, *Untold Stories of the ER*, *Mystery Diagnosis*, *Ask a Mortician*.

Our friends and family know this about us, which I guess is why most of them feel at liberty to turn our cell phones into minefields of unsolicited pics of genitals, rashes, hemorrhoids, or pieces of toilet paper with mystery secretions on them. The questions that accompany these images usually fall along the lines of, "Should this [limb/orifice/sexual organ] look like this?"

I've seen so many things that I wish I hadn't! Because here's the thing: the reason all those YouTube surgery videos don't gross us out is because there's a level of separation. The people in them are *strangers*.

Knowing that a festering wound or mysterious fluid is attached to your best friend changes everything. (To any friends reading this: I don't mind helping you diagnose your problem, and I LOVE YOU DEARLY, but I prefer that you hold off on the pics and use words to describe your condition first. Or at least give me a warning. Pretty please?) Separation is what allows us to do our jobs with objectivity and calm.

Which is why nursing on the fly is so hard with your own children. I remember the look of shock on Jordan's face when he watched me reach over and calmly flick across the room a piece of strawberry that had been trapped in the throat of our two-year-old niece, Aliyah. Aliyah is family, but I had also just come off a night shift in labour and delivery and was basically still in automaton mode.

Even I find it hard to square that response with another one I gave on an evening two years earlier, when our eight-year-old son Logan, who is deathly allergic to nuts, managed to get peanut butter on his hands. (Possibly this was related, ahem, to a peanut butter sandwich Jordan had made for himself and then left the plate lying around. But I can't be sure.)

We scrubbed Logan's hands and put him to bed, but a short time later he came downstairs. He was calm, despite looking like he'd been stung by a thousand bees. One side of his face was completely swollen, and his tongue was so thick he couldn't talk.

When I saw him, I lost my shit; I began to cry and became almost hysterical. I gave Logan some Benadryl and called 911. When the medics arrived, the first thing they asked was whether I had given him an EpiPen.

At the time this event took place, I was working in maternal/child as an educator, where I dealt with reactions like Logan's on a daily basis. I knew all the steps to take (as did Jordan). But panic had caused us both to completely forget about the existence of EpiPens. After receiving the epinephrine, Logan had the thrill of riding in the ambulance to the hospital, where they kept him under observation for about five hours to ensure he didn't experience any negative reactions to the drug.

When we finally got home late at night, he was in good shape. Significantly better than I was! Guilt can really do a number on your brain. I felt embarrassed and humiliated. How could it be that I was able to react one way—the correct way—for another person's child but not my own? Instead of nursing on the fly when I needed to most, in my own field of specialty no less, I'd seen all my hard-won nursing knowledge fly out the window.

WHEN I THINK about all the times I've successfully nursed on the fly, the story that always comes to mind is the one about the patient I had to nurse while, quite literally, flying.

I was working in labour and delivery at a hospital with a 2C level of care (Level 1 being the lowest, except in the US, where the rankings are flipped), which meant we took uncomplicated low-medium risk pregnancies over 30 weeks. I'd been on the job just short of a year, so I wasn't quite a "baby nurse," but I was still a bright-eyed, bushy-tailed, interested-in-everything-and-asking-a-lot-of-questions nurse.

On this particular day I was working triage alongside a more experienced nurse. The patient, a white woman in her mid-thirties named Jowita, had come to us at around 23 weeks into her pregnancy with an incompetent cervix—that is, a cervix that wouldn't stay closed. She had already had multiple miscarriages due to the condition. She'd been treated up to that point by a Level-3 hospital downtown, but she was experiencing some light bleeding and our hospital was the closest.

Jowita's pregnancy was just short of viability, which at this point was considered to be 24 weeks. (Nowadays 23 weeks is viable, and there's talk of dropping the limit to 21 weeks, which I find astounding.)

Jowita's cervix had been stitched closed, a standard treatment for her condition. Her physician would remove the sutures as the true trimester date approached. But when we went to check her, the stitches were gone. In addition, she was starting to experience contractions.

Jowita would have to be transferred to a facility that could handle her now-urgent condition via Ornge, the province's critical-care air ambulance service. While preparations were quickly being made, she was given a sublingual spray of nitro to stop her contractions and hopefully stabilize her situation for the transfer.

My job was to get the necessary charting done to release her. After that, I figured I'd get maybe one more patient before the night was over.

The triage nurse had a different idea. "Amie?" I looked up. "You're going with her."

I scanned the area for other possible Amies, but saw no one.

"Me?! Are you sure?"

I was still too green to know that critical-care patients aren't just handed over to air ambulance staff. They have to be accompanied by someone from the discharging hospital. And because there's often only one doctor on call, that person is usually a nurse.

They called our centre the Birth Factory due to the sheer number of births we handled on a weekly basis, so even though I'd been on the job only a year, I'd managed to gain more expertise than other nurses in a less busy facility. But more importantly in the eyes of my nurse, I was there and I was available.

My initial feeling of excitement—I was being sent on an important mission!—quickly turned to trepidation and unease. The best part about working with a team is that there's always someone to back you up, to turn to for knowledge or an extra set of hands. In emerg, just pressing a button will bring a veritable crowd of staff running towards you.

For this critical transfer, however, I wouldn't just be in charge; I'd be the most experienced person in the room (that room being a helicopter). And did I mention that I hate flying?

As I've said before, nursing culture is sink or swim. This, I could see, was going to be one of those nights when there was a lot of swimming. It was irrelevant that I didn't feel equipped to handle the situation; it was going to happen anyway.

When the air ambulance arrived around 1 a.m., Jowita was understandably freaked out, so I focused on acting calm (I wasn't) and reassuring. I did my best to answer the many questions she threw my way.

The nearest Level 3 hospital was Sunnybrook, just a skip and a jump away, 40 minutes max, but they had no availability. The backup was Ottawa, a full two-hour flight. Due to the helicopter's extremely limited capacity—once the stretcher was inside, it could fit just two EMS staff plus the pilot and me—Jowita's family were not able to accompany her, so her nervous father jumped in the car and said he'd meet us in Ottawa.

THE DECEMBER NIGHT was snowy and windswept as we wheeled Jowita to the chopper. I was to sit behind her head while one medic sat next to me, the other up front with the pilot. As we strapped in for lift-off, it was hard to shake a sense of impending doom.

Once we were airborne, however, my terror was mitigated somewhat by the fact that I had to perform labour and delivery assessments on Jowita every fifteen minutes. This included checking for bleeding and monitoring her blood pressure, heart, and respiration, the frequency of her contractions (which she was still experiencing, despite the nitro), and the firmness of her cervix.

I kept my exams external to avoid stimulating the cervix and activating labour. But a lot of my focus was on trying to keep her comfortable. I haven't held the hands of many patients during my career, but with Jowita it felt like the right thing to do.

She kept asking me if I thought her baby was going to make it or if she was going to deliver during the flight. I wanted to comfort her, but I told her honestly that I couldn't predict these things.

My biggest fear was that I'd have to deliver the baby in that flying tin can with none of the usual resources. If she had a heart attack, then the EMS were on hand. But what if she had a postpartum hemorrhage or some other complication? Once again, it made me appreciate working as part of a team.

But I was not willing to engage in a conversation about such worst-case scenarios. I had seen the pain and sadness of a woman forced to deliver a stillborn baby at 20 weeks, so I tried to keep the mood upbeat and inspire a confidence in Jowita that I didn't truly feel myself.

"We're getting you to the right place," I kept saying. I also used my other soft skills: distracting her, talking about family, even telling a few jokes.

When we landed in Ottawa around 3 a.m., Jowita's baby was still inside her. I wished her the best as she disappeared through the hospital's swinging doors. A half-hour later, I handed off my final report, reassured knowing that she was in the best possible hands.

The medics I flew with had told me that, provided they didn't get another call, they could take me back to Toronto. I was loading my jacket, stethoscope, lunch bag, and chart back into the aircraft when that call came in.

Minutes later I was standing alone in a big, dark field behind the hospital as my ride took off without me. I walked slowly back to the hospital, unsure how I was supposed to get home by myself in the middle of the night. I didn't even have a cell phone, so I couldn't call Jordan to ask him what to do.

Technically, I was also still on shift. At 4 a.m., after a round of desperate calls on the hospital phones, I found a cab willing to undertake the four-hour drive to Toronto. I finally walked through the doors of my hospital at 8:30 a.m. Before going home, I needed to hand in my report and sign out. A colleague spotted me. "How was your shift?" she asked cheerfully.

The whole experience had been physically and emotionally exhausting. So exhausting that when I finally got home, I couldn't sleep. After that, I made it my mission to avoid air transfers. In the future, I decided, all my nursing would be done on solid ground!

NURSE *WITH* GRIT

Sheilabye (Sheila) Sobrany (b. 1969)

Sheilabye Sobrany called her first few weeks as president of the Royal College of Nurses a baptism by fire. Not only was the UK's main nursing union about to embark on the biggest strike in its 106-year history in response to falling pay and understaffing, but a recent report had found the RCN itself to be plagued with misogyny, sexual harassment, bullying, racism, and other forms of dysfunction. Sobrany had come to the position following a long career as a nurse and nurse educator. At Middlesex University, where she was a lecturer, she founded the school's Anti-Racism Network, as well as several other anti-racism groups. As incoming RCN president, she made it clear that anti-racism, as well as fair pay, would be the top concerns. "Everybody needs to be on board with cultural changes," she told a reporter. "I wanted to bring that here into this role, and that's the reason I put myself forward as president."

Lindsay Pentland

Travel nursing isn't as lucrative in Canada as it is in the US, but it still attracts a lot of people who want to get away from the grind of full-time bedside nursing. For fourteen years, registered practical nurse Lindsay Pentland was mostly happy with her job at a small hospital in the town of Leamington, Ontario, a one-hour drive to Detroit on Lake Erie. Fast-forward to 2021: like so many nurses, she was experiencing total burnout and ready to quit the profession she loved without a Plan B. (Lindsay actually has a problem with the word *burnout*. What nurses were asked to do during Covid, she says, went against the morals most had been raised with.) She credits travel nursing with saving her mind and her career.

Lindsay, who's in her mid-thirties, grew up in Tecumseh, Ontario, a small town near Windsor. Severe allergies killed her first dream of becoming a vet, but she still wanted to work in the medical field, so nursing seemed like a good fallback. Leamington was her first placement in nursing school, and although she was only making beds and bathing patients, she was struck by the "phenomenal" group of nurses there. She went to nearby Windsor for the rest of her clinical consolidations, but Leamington stuck with her, so much so that when a job came up she was willing to drive an extra 45 minutes to take it. Eventually, she bought a house with the idea of settling there permanently.

Like Nurse Q, Lindsay first learned about travel nursing in college. It sounded like something she might want to do, but at the time they didn't hire RPNs. (The difference between RNs and RPNs comes down to education. While both are taught from the same body of nursing knowledge, RNs study for a longer period of time, allowing for a greater depth and breadth of foundational knowledge and expanded scope of practice. At the end of the day, though, both are nurses!) By 2016, this had changed, so she submitted her application to a travel nurse agency. They were only placing clients in nursing and retirement homes. That wasn't her thing, so she let it go.

LINDSAY HAS WORKED in most areas of Leamington's fifty-eight-bed hospital. You name it: acute, palliative, ambulatory, med-surg, rehab, Covid response, stabilization. She's also worked at a pain clinic. When the pandemic hit, she was in the Rapid Assessment Zone (RAZ), where they took care of Levels 3-5 in the triage system (Level 1 being the most acute). As an RPN, she often worked alongside a nurse practitioner and a doctor, with the three bouncing back and forth and covering for one another as needed. Remember we said there is an ER type? That's Lindsay. Physically restless ("I can't sit still!"), she thrives on the craziness, the constant change, the not knowing from day to day what she'll get. With Covid, however, she hit her limit.

Thinking back to 2020, Lindsay recalls turning to a colleague and simply saying, "We're fucked." A unique set of circumstances made Leamington the last place in Ontario to recover from the pandemic's first wave—which, for the community of 27,000, was actually three mini-waves. The first wave was comprised of long-term–care patients. The second included migrant workers, thousands of whom come to Leamington, Canada's greenhouse capital, from Mexico every summer to work in agriculture. The third wave afflicted the area's substantial Mennonite population, which continued attending church when the rest of the country was avoiding socializing. The virus had a field day. Many of the Mennonites Lindsay saw in the ER spoke no English, just Low German, one of the few languages not offered through the hospital's translation phone line. Since patients' inability to communicate was adding to an already stressful situation, the hospital obtained a bunch of iPads so that relatives could help with translation and, in some cases, say their final goodbyes. (Instituting the use of iPads for patient care and communication was one of the few good things to come out of the pandemic, Lindsay maintains.)

The craziness she had once embraced as an ER nurse became untenable during Covid. "I lost sight of the care in our healthcare system as I saw the way everyone was being treated, from patients to staff to employers." Friends told her, "You haven't been yourself for a year." In January 2021, Lindsay called her accountant and asked if she had enough money to quit her job. He went through her finances and told her she might be okay . . . for a little while.

The skill set required of RPNs like Lindsay had increased dramatically over the years. Salaries, on the other hand, had not followed suit. A couple of other incidents further drove home the conviction that her profession was treating her less than fairly. In August 2021, a hydrogen sulphide leak caused an explosion under a bar close to Lindsay's home, obliterating the bar and the building next door and forcing local residents to evacuate. As soon as Lindsay heard the ear-shattering noise, she ran over to help. Upon arrival, she found paramedics and firefighters already moving around the chaotic scene, treating victims. A base had been set up at the side of the road with ambulances parked synchronously so that medics could treat victims in an orderly manner.

After all the victims had been either treated and released or sent to hospital, as hoses sprayed the smouldering debris, Lindsay watched in amazement as EMS officers turned their attention to their own. She saw a medic being pulled aside by her chief. "You'll be taking tomorrow off," he said. He was telling her, not asking her. One paramedic even asked Lindsay how she was.

Despite the profound psychological and emotional stresses Lindsay and her colleagues experienced on a daily basis, no such care model existed for nurses.

At one point, Lindsay ended up in her own hospital's ER after someone she knew attacked her. The next day, she told her manager something bad had happened to her and asked if she could go home early. She didn't go into detail about the incident or mention that she'd charged her assailant with assault. It was a small hospital and word got around, so she figured she didn't need to.

Although Lindsay's manager was a social worker by training, she didn't ask Lindsay any further questions. The day was a slow one; on these days nurses are sometimes given the option to go home. But the manager didn't bother to check in with the charge nurse to see how busy things were. She simply declined Lindsay's request.

Lindsay didn't push back. Although she had been at the hospital over a decade, this was her first week working in the ER and she didn't want to look bad or let her colleagues down. During her break, she arranged for a friend to be at her house when the locksmith arrived to change the locks.

INCIDENTS LIKE THESE were piling up for Lindsay. So in June 2021, when the travel nurse agency called her out of the blue and asked her to update her profile, she was happy to do so. "It felt like the universe was smacking me in the face and saying, *This* is what you want to do," she says. Contract offers quickly followed. Lindsay was given five destinations to choose from in Ontario and British Columbia. Working in BC was appealing, but it required obtaining a $500 licence, so she opted to stay in Ontario.

Four days after the explosion, she was on a Thunder Air flight to Fort Albany First Nation, a fly-in reserve in James Bay, Ontario. Centuries earlier, it had been one of the Hudson's Bay Company's key outposts. Lindsay had been north before, in places like Sault Ste. Marie on Lake Superior, but this was the *true* north. From Leamington, as the crow flies (or the plane—there are no roads leading there), Fort Albany is almost half the distance to BC, even though they're both in the same province.

Lindsay knew right away that she was going to love the place. If Leamington was small, the hospital in Fort Albany was tiny: fourteen beds, nine of which were taken up by continuing-care patients. The ER consisted of one trauma room, one hold room, and two exam rooms. The hospital had no lab techs or even in-house doctors, and most of the nurses were travellers like Lindsay. Nurses did all blood draws and EKGs. There were no Covid patients, at least not until Lindsay's last day.

First Nations reserves often make headlines for what's wrong with them, whether it's boil-water advisories or social problems like addiction, which are often related to Canada's history of colonialism and residential schools (Fort Albany's reserve had the reputation of being one of the worst), so Lindsay was pleased to see that most of the hospital's full-time staff, including the X-ray technician and ward clerks, were Indigenous. Arriving in August for a six-week contract, she got to spend Thanksgiving and the first National Day for Truth and

Reconciliation there. Despite some obvious challenges, Fort Albany struck Lindsay as a tight, deeply grounded community full of strong, generous people.

An example of this generosity was illustrated shortly after she stepped off the plane. Due to Covid, Lindsay would have to quarantine before entering the community, so she'd brought along a week's worth of food, including a cooler full of meat that had gone missing in transit. Upon hearing this, the hospital's cook immediately stepped up to make Lindsay meals, sneaking extra food for her to take home. And the food, which was the same as what the patients ate, was *delicious*. Ribs twice a week!

Shows of kindness continued after her quarantine was over. One of Lindsay's long-term–care patients taught her Cree, which she then practised on another LTC patient who had once been the Cree teacher for the entire community. When Lindsay spoke to her she lit up, thrilled that this white girl from down south was making an honest effort to speak the local language.

Her time in Fort Albany was so amazing that when she got the opportunity to return in February 2022 for another five-week stint, Lindsay didn't hesitate. And though the Covid risk was now higher, her experience was just as positive, if not more so. She got to drive on ice roads and see the northern lights for the first time.

But the highlight was an invitation to attend a full-moon ceremony in which local women (no men are allowed) shared stories. At the ceremony (where the group accommodated Lindsay by speaking more English than they normally would), she heard things she found difficult to process. One woman who was Lindsay's age had been in residential school until grade 4 (shockingly, the residential school system in Canada wasn't shut down until the 1990s) and her stories were harrowing. After the main ceremony, which was held indoors, the group moved outside to make offerings over a fire. Lindsay already had deep respect for these women's resilience before the ceremony, but she came away from it with even more.

Fort Albany reinvigorated her, reminding her why she went into nursing in the first place. It allowed her, for what felt like the first time, to care for people the way she'd been taught to in nursing school.

While for some nurses the allure of travel nursing is almost entirely monetary, Lindsay's motivation is experience. Her goal is to go to as many places as she can for as long as she can. (The money isn't bad either. Licensing differences between provinces mean that she's sometimes paid more for doing less.)

Like Nurse Q, Lindsay could maximize her earnings by finding a cheaper place to stay and pocket the difference in her stipend. But the agency's turnkey service (it books her plane tickets, her hotel, her shuttle) is a big part of why she loves travel nursing. In Terrace, BC, she stayed for a month in a beautiful hotel with a sauna and hot tub, visited hot springs, and hiked the Nass Valley. In Victoria, she had a breathtaking view of Portage Inlet.

Listening to Lindsay, it seems that nursing agency websites aren't exaggerating their promise of glamorous adventure. For her thirty-sixth birthday, she went to Tofino, on Vancouver Island's stunning Pacific Rim, and spent the whole day surfing. Adventures aside, she has also made new friends, not to mention the crazy, small-town connections that only seem to happen in a country as big, and as small, as Canada. Lindsay grins ear to ear as she describes these experiences as if she can't believe they happened to her: "There are days when I have to remind myself I'm a nurse, not a celebrity."

IN THE SAME VEIN (NURSING ON THE FLY)

Sara

A lot of people assume that when you're a nurse, you've got your nursing hat on 24/7. And in some ways, it's true. Nursing has made me compulsively observant in ways I never was before. For example, I don't look at veins in the way I did in my pre-nursing life, if I even looked at them at all back then. I can't tell you the number of times I've found myself in a lineup at Costco or Ikea staring at the veiny arms of the person in front of me, thinking, "That would be a nice, easy one. . . " This unconscious habit is way worse in summer when people are in short sleeves. When Amie and I met Prime Minister Justin Trudeau at the International Council for Nurses Congress, my eyes quickly slipped down to his hands. Think what you want of his politics, but he has excellent veins.

My kids are aware of my vein obsession, having been at the receiving end of it since they were born. I'll point to the back of their hands and say, "Look at this juicy one . . . it's really straight, so if you ever go to the hospital, they'll put the needle right *there*."

In addition to staring at people's veins in stores, I've also caught myself looking up at the night sky during a full moon, wondering how busy the emergency and maternity units are (many healthcare providers have anecdotally provided a correlation between a full moon and situations such as unexpected labour and worsening psychiatric symptoms).

I want to be clear: There are no intentions or judgment behind any of these thoughts. I would never go up to a stranger and comment on their gator veins, although I admit I have told people I know who seem shaky and irritable when they're hungry that they might have hypoglycemia. In fact, at one point I had so many symptoms of hypoglycemia I thought I had it myself. (My blood-sugar test was negative. Apparently I just have a low tolerance for hunger, which isn't great when your job involves working 12-hour shifts!)

And while there are times when, for sanity's sake, we nurses really need to take our professional glasses off completely, a lot of the time it feels like they're just sitting on top of our heads, waiting to fall back down. The classic dilemma is what to do when you witness an accident while off-shift. At school they taught us that we don't *have* to get involved, but if we do we have to follow through. In other words, you can't start treating someone and then decide you don't want to miss the trailers at that movie you were on your way to see and abandon the victim in the middle of the process.

Nursing on the fly can happen in all kinds of unexpected places— even hospitals. Take the time I was working in postpartum and my patient's husband collapsed. (I learned after the fact that he was an alcoholic who had decided to detox after the birth of his child. This was admirable, but he decided to do it on his own, cold turkey.) We were in the mother's room when he fell, hitting his head hard. He lay on the floor, completely unconscious. There was so much blood around him it was hard to tell where it was coming from. As I bent down to have a look, I caught a strong whiff of alcohol from his breath. Apparently the detox hadn't lasted long.

I glanced at the mother, who was holding her newborn and looking at her prone and bleeding husband with a calmness that told me she'd seen this happen before. But she had recently delivered by C-section, so she couldn't be of much help to me.

Because the mom was my patient, not her husband, I had to treat him as if I were a first responder, so I pressed the Code Blue button (although he technically still had vital signs, he was unconscious and required immediate help). The usual protocol after calling a Code Blue is to step back and wait until the Code Blue team arrives, but I didn't feel I could just stand there. Therefore, while telling myself that the man's condition could have a profound effect on my patient's wellbeing, I wiped up the small pool of blood that had formed next to his head and continued to check his vitals. I felt a pulse and could see his chest rising. Phew.

Seconds later, a few of my co-workers rushed in. They pushed the bed against the wall to make room for the group of ten+ team members behind them. I stood by my patient, explaining what was happening and reassuring her while the team tended to her husband. (Later, a social worker came by to make sure she was okay.) They got him to sit up and started an IV and applied Steri-Strips on the cut to his head before moving him to a wheelchair. He revived quickly, only to lose consciousness again. They transferred him to the emergency department for observation, but by the time I came back for my next shift my patient had gone home, so I never learned her husband's fate, although I have to assume it was a positive one.

NURSING ON THE fly sometimes means making a call that isn't in your job description, or that feels uncomfortable, but is completely necessary in the moment. Once when I was working in a gynecology clinic, I had to stop a very well-respected physician (he delivered celebrities' babies) from using a medical instrument that hadn't been properly sterilized. The patient was there for a follow-up after receiving abnormal results from a routine pap smear. Like many women, she found the procedure painful, so she had asked for it to be done with a smaller speculum. There was only one of those in the clinic. It had already been used that morning and was sitting in a bin awaiting sterilization. The doctor saw the speculum in the bin and said to me nonchalantly, "We'll just wash it off with cleaning solution."

"We *can't* do that!" I said, appalled.

At this point I'd only been a nurse for a couple of years and had never spoken to a doctor so boldly (nowadays I wouldn't hesitate). But this was a bridge too far. There's no "three-second rule" in healthcare. Instruments *have* to be sterilized properly with chemicals in an autoclave. That poor woman could have contracted an STI or a bacterial or viral infection!

Knowing he didn't have a leg to stand on, the doctor quickly backtracked, declaring that we didn't have a small speculum and we would simply use the bigger one, as if that had been his intention all along. All this time the woman had been lying on the table, unaware of our tense exchange. I prayed she hadn't heard what I had said to him.

EVEN IF WE don't identify as round-the-clock nurses, some people may still see us that way. It's considered bad form to ask a doctor for medical advice at a cocktail party, but no such etiquette seems to exist when it comes to nurses. Family, friends, and even strangers ask me all kinds of questions at any time. How to find a family doctor, whether my hospital is hiring, what the strange rash on their neck is. For the most part I don't mind, but there are times when I need to draw the line—like when I got a message on LinkedIn from a stranger asking me what to do about the mole on her mother's back!

During the pandemic, people couldn't get enough of talking about Covid, especially regarding their frustration with vaccinations in the early rollouts. Given the intensity of the situation, I was usually happy to engage in these conversations, especially if it meant correcting misinformation. I've always had a hard time with non-scientific, "holistic" approaches to health. They just don't resonate with me. My general thinking is this: if you have a viral infection and you think you can cure it with an herbal product, go ahead and try, but don't take liberties fooling around with other people's health. I've seen children die of meningitis because parents didn't take their symptoms seriously or used unproven home remedies to treat it. Sometimes people refuse to talk to me once they realize I disagree with their flaky opinions. I'm fine with this; we don't have to agree to get along. For instance, I still talk to my anti-vax neighbour as long as we stick to safe topics like pop culture, travel, or food (I'm a *big* foodie).

The most frequent requests I get are about navigating the healthcare system. What bothers me here isn't the request itself; it's the term *navigate*. I believe that in a public system no one should have to do this.

I THINK A lot of nurses would agree that nursing on the fly is hardest, and weirdest, when it involves family. I recall the day in December 2022 when I found myself confronting a potentially dire medical situation affecting our seven-year-old son, James.

My husband, Kevin, and I woke up that morning to a strange shuffling that was slowly making its way to our bedroom. The sound stopped, the door opened, and James shuffled over to the bed on his knees.

"Get up," I told him, assuming he was being silly.

"I can't," he said matter-of-factly.

James is a kid who loves to fool us and joke around, but I wasn't yet in the mood for games (he can also be a little lazy, which is what the shuffling seemed like). Ignoring him, I got up and got on with my day.

Twenty minutes later, however, he was still "kneeing" around the house.

"Let me help you," I said, thinking that playing along would make the game end faster. But as I lifted James up from under the armpits, I felt his legs buckle beneath me like a rag doll.

This didn't feel like a game anymore. I let my nursing goggles fall on my nose: could it be growing pains?

I bent down to be at eye level with James. "Do your legs hurt?"

"No, I just can't walk. They feel like jelly."

It was a weekend and there was no rush to go anywhere, so James spent most of the day on his iPad. When he needed to get somewhere, he shuffled over on his knees. To be honest, I wasn't paying complete attention. I still wasn't convinced that he wasn't play-acting. And it definitely didn't seem like a medical issue. He wasn't in pain and he didn't have any other symptoms. I'm a person who tries hard not to overreact. I figured that giving him time and space would surely make whatever it was go away.

Kevin wasn't so convinced. He's a worrier, and as the day went on with no change in James's condition he started googling. Then came the armchair diagnosis: Guillain-Barré syndrome (GBS), a rare and serious condition in which the immune system attacks healthy nerve cells, resulting in weakness in the legs, difficulty walking, and, in some cases, paralysis. GBS, Kevin read, can be brought on by an infectious illness. At this point we both stopped and looked at each other. The whole family had just had a bout of cold and flu-like symptoms.

It was 9 p.m., too late to get to a doctor. It was also James's bedtime, so I suggested we simply go to the local walk-in clinic the next day. Kevin, like me, is calm and rational about most things, except when it comes to health stuff. By now he was in a full-blown, tearful panic. And I could see that our opposing reactions seemed to be negatively affecting James's mental state. So when Kevin announced that he was taking him to emerg, I didn't even try to stop him.

When he was at the hospital, Kevin realized that his phone was dying. He didn't have a charger, so he didn't send un update until almost midnight: "Done bloodwork, started IV, pain meds. In middle of EKG."

All good. But then came another message shortly after the first: James had been diagnosed with myocarditis, an inflammation of the heart that was strongly associated with Covid.

I texted back: "Do the nurses and doctors look stressed?" but got no response. It was now after midnight, so Kevin's phone was probably dead. I thought I might as well go to sleep.

But before turning in for the night, I did some quick googling of my own and discovered that although myocarditis wasn't at the level of Guillain-Barré, it was still pretty serious. Now I was the one freaking out. Had my failure to recognize symptoms of a serious disease put our son in peril?

I woke up briefly when Kevin and James walked through the door at 2 a.m., but they went to sleep in a different part of the house. If James's condition was really serious, I reasoned in my hazy state, then surely Kevin would have come and told me. Also, they would not have sent him home. (I shut out the fact that this was also a time of extreme staff shortages. I'd just read about a woman who died in the ER after coming in with abdominal pains because no one took her seriously.)

In the morning, Kevin explained that his text had contained a typo. James didn't have myocarditis; he had *myositis*, a rare but benign childhood muscle condition. Elevated enzyme levels in his blood related to muscle breakdown had confirmed it. There was nothing to be done except encourage him to drink lots of fluids to flush out the enzyme (which, in extremely rare cases, could cause kidney damage). Left untreated, the condition usually resolves itself in a matter of days. The outcome would have been the same whether Kevin had taken James to the hospital or not.

To prevent James from wearing out the knees of his pants, we gave him an office chair with wheels and had some fun pushing him around the house. Later that week, I met another mom whose kid had had the condition twice and was fine. This was a huge relief.

But it did make me reflect on how my and Kevin's personalities had affected how the whole thing played out. Admittedly, the myocarditis text had worried me, but not enough to keep me awake. Kevin, on the other hand, is an engineer trained to consider worst-case scenarios, which is exactly where his head went until he finally got the all-clear.

When we went to our family doctor's office for a follow-up, we saw a nurse practitioner. Clearly at a loss about what to do, she sent us for bloodwork, which we didn't complete because James is terrified of needles. This wasn't a nursing call, it was a mom call, and it turned out to be the right one. Three days later, James had abandoned his wheelie chair and was running around as if nothing ever happened.

NURSE[S] WITH GRIT

Amie Archibald-Varley (b. 1984)
and Sara Fung (b. 1985)

As nurses, we're taught to be humble. To be okay with the modifier "*only* a nurse." But if nursing is going to evolve, we need to start taking credit for the important work we do. To toot our own horns. Because unless you're Florence Nightingale, no one's going to toot it for you. So it's in this spirit that we're putting ourselves on this list.

We created *The Gritty Nurse Podcast* out of what felt like necessity, with no idea where it would take us. It was the early days of the pandemic, and the difference between the hero treatment nurses were getting in the media and the brutal reality of our actual workplaces couldn't have been more stark. Covid-19 was being politicized in mind-boggling ways, and it still is to this day. Hoping to make sense of it all, and to feel less alone, we started having conversations with an eclectic mix of people—physicians, authors, patient advocates, mental health advocates. We wanted to build community and get our voices heard, help the public understand our struggles at the bedside, understand that nursing and healthcare are inherently political, that nursing can be a force for positive social change. If just one person listened to us and thought, "Hey, that's my experience too"—which they did, time and again—it feels revolutionary to us. So, icky as it feels to put ourselves here, we're doing it anyway!

The Case of RaDonda Vaught

O*n a May morning* in 2022, hundreds of nurses gathered from across the US outside a Nashville, Tennessee, courthouse. They held signs with slogans like "Nurses are NOT criminals!" and "Yesterday's HERO, today's SCAPEGOAT!" and "To err is human, unless you're a nurse. Then it's CRIMINAL."

They were there for the sentencing of RaDonda Vaught, a nurse from Vanderbilt University Medical Center. In March, Vaught had been convicted of criminally negligent homicide and gross neglect of an impaired adult. In 2017, she had accidentally administered the incorrect medication to a patient. (She had been found not guilty of the more serious charge of reckless homicide.)

The nurses were there to support Vaught. As the "#IAmRadonda" hashtag on the T-shirts they were wearing indicated, every nurse who was there knew that they could have been the one convicted of the same "crimes."

VAUGHT HAD BEEN practising nursing for two years without incident. In fact, as doctors would testify at her trial, she was in most regards the ideal nurse, dedicated and reliable. The victim, seventy-five-year-old Charlene Murphey, was not Vaught's patient. Vaught was simply doing her part to help her busy colleagues in an all-hands-on-deck situation.

Murphey, who was suffering from a brain bleed, was scheduled for a PET scan. Due to her debilitating claustrophobia, she required sedation before entering the confining PET machine. Vaught had been told to administer Versed. But when she entered the name of the sedative into the hospital's automatic medication dispenser, nothing showed up. Assuming this was yet another software issue, Vaught performed a manual override that would allow her to access stronger medications. She typed in "VE" again and selected the first drug that was suggested to her: vecuronium, a powerful paralytic given to patients undergoing surgery to ensure they don't move around on the operating table.

Despite a boldfaced label on the container that read "Warning: Paralyzing Agent," Vaught injected the patient with the drug. Then she placed Murphey's gurney in the hallway outside the PET scan room. Shortly afterwards, Charlene Murphey stopped breathing. (Had she received Versed, the milder drug she was supposed to get—which turned out to be listed under its generic name, midazolam—leaving her alone would have been acceptable practice.)

The next day, Murphey died.

Profoundly distraught, RaDonda Vaught didn't try to deflect the blame for what she had done. Following the incident, she willingly answered various investigators' questions with no attorney present. No one read her rights to her.

The Vanderbilt Medical Center let Vaught go, but it didn't disclose her error to state or federal regulators as legally required. Instead, the hospital told the local medical examiner's office that Murphey had died of natural causes. The hospital reached a settlement with Charlene

Murphey's family, part of which was an agreement not to discuss the cause of her death in public (which at that point the family wasn't even aware of). It made no changes to its protocols, even though Charlene Murphey's death clearly involved systemic as well as human error. In the meantime, Vaught found employment elsewhere.

Charlene Murphey's family learned the truth about the medication error a year and a half later from an anonymous tipster. But although a probe by the Tennessee Bureau of Investigation found that Vanderbilt had covered up its wrongdoing and therefore bore a "heavy burden of responsibility" in Murphey's death, the state's health department chose not to hold the hospital accountable.

Instead, with the incident now in the public eye, it set its sights on Vaught.

In July 2021, a tearful Vaught gave testimony in front of the Tennessee Board of Nursing in which she admitted the mistake was "completely my fault." Her nursing licence was revoked.

A criminal indictment followed, led by the state's zealous district attorney, Glenn Funk, despite accusations of several conflicts of interest. If convicted of the most serious charges, Vaught faced up to twelve years in prison.

The case was unusual in a number of disturbing ways. Unintentional medical deaths usually go through the civil system or through licensing boards, where the goal is to seek compensation. A *criminal* charge against a nurse for a medical error, where the goal is punishment, was virtually unheard of. It was especially bizarre given that prosecutors weren't claiming Vaught had ever intended to kill Charlene Murphey.

On March 25, 2022, thirty-eight-year-old Vaught was found guilty of the lesser charge: negligent homicide and abuse of an impaired adult. But she still faced jail time. It was an incredibly dark moment for everyone involved: Vaught, Murphey's family, and nurses everywhere.

Then a remarkable thing happened. Nurses started to rally for

Vaught's cause. They posted on social media and attended protests. They flooded the court assigned to her case with emails, voicemails, and letters. They wrote petitions for clemency that received hundreds of thousands of signatures. They got *loud*. A private Facebook group called Nurses March for RaDonda's Law—whose stated aim was to "create a community of people willing to advocate for legislation that will protect healthcare professionals from being prosecuted criminally for making good-faith medical errors"—attracted tens of thousands of members.

On sentencing day, the nurses who gathered in front of the Tennessee courthouse started by taking a minute of silence for Charlene Murphey. No one, including Vaught, was under any illusions about who was the ultimate victim in the unfortunate case.

But when the news was announced that Vaught would get three years' community service but no jail time, cheers erupted throughout the crowd. Many people believe the outcome would have been very different were it not for huge amount of support she received from healthcare workers.

RADONDA VAUGHT'S CASE is horrifying to us for many reasons, not the least of which is the reality that each and every nurse—whether they admit it or not—has made mistakes. We've both given patients incorrect doses of high-alert drugs: morphine (Sara), and insulin (Amie). Luckily, neither dose was sufficiently high to be lethal, but we were both reluctant to disclose what we did out of fear the gavel would come down on us personally.

Criminalizing such errors, however, is another thing entirely. Imagine the chilling effect it would have had on nurses owning up to future mistakes if RaDonda Vaught had been sent to prison? It would certainly scare people away from the profession and in doing so ironically perpetuate the very conditions—understaffing—that contributed to her error in the first place.

Activism is still relatively new to nursing, but it's become clear our place is no longer just at the bedside. We also need to speak out when we see our patients, and each other, put at risk.

Tragic as it was, RaDonda Vaught's case was that rare instance of nurses finding solidarity to advocate for each other. Best of all, we showed that doing this works.

We don't have to be nurse heroes to make a difference. We can each contribute in our own way. Our profession is 20 million strong across the globe, and yet we don't always realize the power we have. Writing a letter to your government representatives can make a difference. Talking to fellow nurses, or friends, about what you can do makes a difference. Speaking up when something happens at the bedside that you know isn't right can make a difference. Marching in a demonstration, whether it's in support of a colleague, or to fight legislation that impacts people's health outcomes, can make a difference. Even a Tweet can make a difference.

To quote Cathy Crowe: "Great nursing happens when the culmination of passion, power, and politics come together in the name of social justice."

THE SISTER (A GHOST STORY)

Matthew Shepherd

I started my nursing career in 2009 in the community setting, but in 2013 I transitioned to the OR. Initially, it was hard to make a connection with people. A patient would get wheeled in, I'd say "Hi," they'd get anaesthetized, then surgery would begin.

My first uncanny experience on the job happened on a night shortly after orientation. Due to a critter problem, the nursing lounge had been moved to an area in an abandoned wing of the hospital that was accessed from the OR by going down two really long hallways.

On this particular night, I was headed to the lounge to get a bite to eat. But as I approached the room, something—or rather some *thing*—compelled me to keep on walking. Feeling curious rather than excited or anxious, I reached a spot where the hall branched in two. On one side was total darkness. On the other, the lights were on in every room. No sooner did I register this fact than all the lights started turning off in sequence, like a motion sensor in reverse.

Freaked out, I ran back to the unit, where I stayed put, hungry but safe. When I shared my experience with a nurse who had been at the hospital for twenty-five years, she was matter of fact. "Ah, you met the Sister," she said. I learned that the Sister had once been a nurse, and as her calling card she went around the hospital turning lights off to save energy. I guess if you're going to haunt a place, you should at least do it for a good cause!

I and some of the other nurses started to have similar experiences in the OR. I'd be in a room doing some task and the light would just turn off (and no, it wasn't on a timer). But again, I never sensed any insidious aura. I should say here that my Jamaican father and Portuguese mother raised me to believe in the spirit world. I'm a good judge of energies, and the ones I've experienced in hospitals were usually positive.

Shortly after I "met" the Sister, things started to happen outside of the hospital. At the time, I had just moved into a new basement apartment. One night after a long shift I was watching TV on the couch when I noticed the hall light become noticeably dim.

When I got up to investigate, I found that the light switch was stuck halfway between on and off, so it was odd. I turned it fully back on and sat down, and then . . . it happened again.

Thinking the light bulb must be malfunctioning, I texted my landlady, who lived upstairs. She came down the next day to check it out and couldn't find a problem, but she changed the bulb anyway (she was a great landlady).

Two days later, again while I was watching TV, the light dimmed in exactly the same way. What I'd previously suspected now seemed certain: this was no malfunction, but rather the work of some meddlesome spirit. My parents had always taught me that the latter should be treated respectfully but assertively, so that's the approach I tried to take. "This is my home. You're not welcome here," I said as firmly as I could. "Leave me alone!"

This seemed to work, at least for a while. It was two weeks before the light dimming happened again. But this time when I got up to turn off the light, there was a new surprise: my front door was wide open. Even more strange, the screen door was closed. I texted my landlady to ask if she had been down to my apartment. She said no.

Since I'd only recently moved in, I asked her if the previous tenant might still have keys.

She doubted this was the case, but out of an abundance of caution she changed the locks anyway (did I mention she was a really good landlady?).

Before going to bed I locked the screen door, the main door deadbolt, and the privacy lock. When I woke up in the morning the door was wide open again. The privacy lock was still secure, but the (brand new) deadbolt was retracted.

The next night at work, I was assigned to help with organ procurement from a young man who had succumbed to his injuries in a motorcycle accident. These are very lengthy procedures and we didn't finish until around 1 a.m. Normally a nurse's aid would take the body to the morgue, but none was available. Probably because I was the only man working that night, the task fell to me and another nurse. The sub-basement where the morgue is located has lots of offices, and during the day it's busy. But at night, it feels like . . . a morgue.

After taking the elevator down, we wheeled the body to the refrigerator cabinet. When I opened the door, the air inside felt unusually cold and intense. I suddenly felt anxious. Working in the OR had made me used to frigid temperatures, but this cold felt cloying, nasty. I had a bad feeling.

But this was the body of someone's beloved and I wanted to be respectful and take my time. We gently and securely placed the corpse with the six others already there and finished by affixing the tag. As we were preparing to close the fridge door, we heard a loud, hard thud.

The other nurse gave up all pretense of calm and screamed, *"It moved!"*

"It can't move, it doesn't have organs!" I screamed back. Had we forgotten to tie the young man's hands together over his stomach as per protocol? I quickly dismissed these doubts. Not only were there two of us there, but also the other nurse was known for dotting her i's and crossing her t's. But at this point neither of us was prepared to investigate the source of the noise. We got out of there as quickly as we could.

When I got home it was still dark, and I felt scared, which was unusual: I've *never* felt scared in my own space. I turned on the TV and started flipping channels in the hopes of finding something that would take my mind off what had happened. And then—you guessed it—the hallway light dimmed again. My fear suddenly turned into annoyance and I yelled at the light, "Stop it! I don't want to deal with you or your friends!" As soon as the words were out of my mouth, the light turned off completely.

I had locked all three locks, this time adding the chain, which I'd never used before. When I woke up the next morning, both doors—entryway and now the screen—were wide open.

I took a photo and sent it to the landlady, who immediately came down. She assured me that she had not come in. Unfortunately, I knew she was telling the truth.

It was hard to shake the feeling that my trip to the morgue had changed something. The insidiousness that I felt when I opened the frigid cabinet and then heard the thump now seemed to be inside my home.

Two nights later the weirdness ramped up. The other lights in my apartment, including the kitchen, started flickering and then went out completely. When I sat in the living room, I felt that I was being watched from the kitchen.

"What do you want? What *is* this?" I yelled. After receiving no response—had I expected one?—I turned off the TV and went to bed.

In the middle of the night, I woke up. Not in the normal, gradual way. Instead, I hinged forward from my hips and sat bolt upright. My bedroom opened onto the living room, and when I looked in that direction I saw the silhouette of a man—although I didn't feel he/it was human—looking back at me. The body itself was darker than the dark, yet I could somehow see through it.

Unlike the feeling earlier in the evening, this wasn't insidious. I didn't feel like this being wanted to hurt me. I tried addressing him/it: "If you're here because you're curious, fine. But I don't want to deal with you." I put my head down and fell asleep again.

Two hours later, I woke up in exactly the same position: bolt upright. I opened my eyes and the figure was at the foot of my bed, staring at me. There was still no sense of malice, just a curious presence in my room. I must have gone back to sleep.

Two hours later I woke again, but I didn't sit bolt upright because the thing was now hovering over me, in my face. I swung my arm at it, screaming, *"Get out! I'm tired of this shit! You're not welcome here in my room. What do you want?"*

At this point the creature simply dissipated.

When I woke up the next day, I wondered if it had all been a dream. But a quick glance at Sleep Cycle, the app I used, proved otherwise. Not only was there a graph showing my sleep and wake cycle but also a recording of all the things I yelled out. The whole night had occurred exactly the way I remembered it.

My sense that this spirit was connected to my work at the hospital was confirmed over the next few days. I would wake up to find my scrubs, which I normally keep in my closet, in strange places: on the couch, on the kitchen floor, even in the garbage.

One evening while sitting on the couch as usual, I felt two distinct energies: one curious, the other insidious. I understood that the former was the one that had come into my room; the latter was the one that had turned off the lights and moved my scrubs. Over time, the curious being seemed to go away, leaving me with the insidious one.

I started sleeping with my bedroom door closed but the bathroom door open. One night I woke up to the sound of footsteps that seemed to be coming from the living room. The floor was laminate, so it made a distinct noise, and I could tell from the pattern of the sound that something was walking slowly in a circle.

When the light of dawn began coming through the bathroom window, I heard the being stir, then stop. Then it started going faster and heavier—*thud thud thud thud*—still in a circle, before it stopped at what sounded like the farthest corner of the apartment. As I sat up, the creature ran towards my closed door and stopped. I got out of bed and grabbed the door handle.

When I opened the door there was no one there, but I could see that the front door was wide open. I looked down. There was dirt on the living room floor, but no footprints.

I gave my kind landlady notice the same day. I'd had enough. Coincidentally, my cousin called later in the afternoon. He was coming from Jamaica in a few days and needed a place to stay. Did I have room? Hell yes, I told him. Desperate for company, and not wanting to scare him off, I made no mention of the recent events. But when he arrived, we shared a bottle of wine and I told him everything. He was dubious. "Girl," he said, "spirits don't exist!"

Of course, that night and the following few nights, nothing happened. No dimming lights, no pacing spirits.

Early in the morning about a week later, my cousin texted me. I was already at work. By any chance had I left the oven door open? he asked. And the fridge door? He told me he'd seen light coming from kitchen and found the fridge door wide open.

A few days later—I was again already at work—my cousin texted again. He said he was coming out of the shower when he saw the front door was open. Assuming I must have come home, he called out to me. I didn't answer, so he had texted me. I had to take a pic of myself to prove that I actually was at work.

No longer doubting my story, he went out and bought some sage for smudging. "I want to respect you," he said to the room as he smudged it. "But you're not welcome here." He did a smudging when I was at home, and another when I wasn't. After that, there were no more incidents. If I had known it was that easy, I would have done it myself!

Two months later, when I moved into my new place, I smudged everywhere pre-emptively. I don't know if that's the reason, but nothing weird ever happened to me there.

Strange things still happen at work, though. Lights turn off spontaneously. Supplies disappear then turn up in odd places, like my locker. As long as it doesn't feel nefarious, I accept such mischief as part of working in a place where people die every day.

Rachel Radyk

"*You're stupid as hell.*"

"Who do you think is paying for this?"

"You made some bad choices. What are your children going to think, seeing you like this?"

"You're only good for sex."

These racist taunts were some of the final words thirty-seven-year-old Joyce Echaquan heard before she died of a pulmonary edema while tied to a bed in a hospital in Joliette, Quebec. They were uttered in French, a language Echaquan did not speak, by nurses who took the erratic behaviour and agonized screaming of the Atikamekw mother of seven to be that of a drug addict in withdrawal. Echaquan was admitted to the hospital on September 28, 2020, with severe stomach pains and given morphine, even though she warned staff that she might have an adverse reaction to it. She was then left unattended. A woman who was at the hospital that night with her ill father—and who happened to be a patient attendant from another facility—was disturbed by Echaquan's

pleas and the reception they were getting from staff. She approached
Echaquan and asked if she could be of any help. Staff told her to mind
her own business.

Later, that same attendant would recognize Echaquan in a Facebook
video that Echaquan herself had livestreamed in the minutes leading
up to her death. The attendant told the press she regretted not following her instincts and reporting what she saw: "No one deserves to be
treated that way in a hospital."

A diabetic who also had a heart condition that required a pacemaker, Echaquan had been a frequent visitor to the Joliette hospital
for six years. She had come to dread the visits because of the way staff
treated her and started recording live videos as a form of protection.
Several members of her family were unaware that Echaquan was even
in hospital until they saw her seven-minute video in real time. When a
nurse realized she was being recorded she tried, unsuccessfully, to take
Echaquan's phone and delete the video. In the end, the video did not
protect Echaquan, but it did help to expose the ongoing racist abuse of
Indigenous people in Canada's healthcare system. Had it not been for
the public furor that followed, Echaquan would have been just another
dead Indigenous woman. A statistic.

A coroner's report would later rule that Echaquan's death was acci-
dental, but it also took pains to note that the "racism and prejudices
that Ms. Echaquan faced certainly contributed to her death." Her death
could almost certainly have been avoided, the report went on, had she
received supervision and cardiac monitoring. The report concluded by
recommending that the Quebec government recognize the existence
of systemic racism in its healthcare system and make commitments to
eliminating it. The report's findings echoed those of the 520-page Viens
report of a year earlier, which found that when it comes to accessing
public services, Indigenous people in Quebec were indisputably victims

of systemic discrimination. The Viens report called for 142 changes in areas ranging from policing to social services to mental health services and even educational curricula.

But Quebec government officials, including Premier François Legault, pushed back. Racism existed, they acknowledged, but not, heaven forbid, *systemic* racism.

As the Viens report, and countless news stories, confirm, what happened to Joyce Echaquan was not an isolated incident. In 2021, Rocky Whitford, a thirty-seven-year-old man from Alexander First Nation in Alberta, took his own life after trying, and failing, to get admitted to a BC hospital three times in a single day while in a state of psychological distress.

In 2020, a nineteen-year-old Indigenous man was released from a Thunder Bay hospital and escorted by hospital security to the shipping and receiving area of a nearby university, where he died a few hours later of suspected suicide. That same year, the government of British Columbia launched an investigation into allegations that healthcare staff at an unnamed hospital liked to play a game called "The Price is Right" where they guessed the blood-alcohol levels of Indigenous patients.

In 2015, it took Michelle Labrecque, an Oneida woman, three visits to a Victoria, BC, hospital to be diagnosed with a broken pelvis. Seven years earlier, Labrecque had gone to the same hospital seeking medication for severe stomach pains. After she disclosed her struggles with alcohol to a doctor, he sent her home with a "prescription" that turned out to be a crude drawing of a beer bottle with a slash through it.

And these are just the stories that make the headlines. Sadly, nursing has a long, well-documented history of perpetuating harm against First Nations people. Some of this was done in colonial institutions like residential schools and Indian hospitals. The latter were established in the early twentieth century under the auspices of controlling outbreaks of disease like tuberculosis and stuck around until the early '80s. As with residential schools, the true goal of these "hospitals" wasn't health but assimilation. This is why, unlike in settler hospitals, the nurses who worked there weren't required to be licensed. "Nursing" is a twisted misnomer for what happened in these institutions, since patients were as likely to be abused as cared for. Survivors describe incidents of forced kissing and isolation, and the use of straitjackets and casts as restraints. Children were physically beaten and fed vomit. Laws put in place in the 1950s that made it a crime for Indigenous people to refuse care or leave Indian hospitals before they were discharged effectively turned them into prisoners.

Nurses didn't just "treat" Indigenous patients in residential schools and Indian hospitals, they also played a pivotal role in getting children *into* these institutions—both before and after the so-called Sixties Scoop—by going into communities and taking them away from their families. Under cover of "public health," nurses were also tasked with creating lists of "undesirable" people, a disproportionate number of whom were Indigenous, to undergo forced sterilization (coerced tubal ligation of Indigenous women was still occurring as recently as 2017). They also conducted bogus "intelligence tests" to identify children with "mental deficiencies" so that they, too, could be sterilized. Taken in combination, these unethical medical practices directly implicate nurses in the epidemic of missing and murdered Indigenous women and girls (MMIWG) in Canada that led to the inquiry of the same name.

Given this shameful history, it's easy to understand why so many First Nations people distrust the healthcare system. For this to change, the healthcare system needs more people like registered nurse and educator Rachel Radyk. An AnishinaabeKwe (Ojibwe woman) in her early thirties with multiple degrees in communications and nursing, Rachel is in a unique position to do what she does: practise trauma-informed care and advocate for Indigenous patients. In addition to working with individuals, Rachel also supports Indigenous and non-Indigenous healthcare organizations in their efforts to combat racism and offer safe spaces for Indigenous clientele.

Before she could help her community, however, Rachel first had to reconnect with it herself. That ongoing journey has been intertwined with her nursing journey in fascinating ways.

Raised Catholic in Ontario's Kitchener-Waterloo area (known by residents as KW), Rachel could never quite shake the feeling that something was missing from her life spiritually. As she got older, she started experimenting with alternative spiritual practices. One practitioner she worked with singled her out for her spirituality. On another occasion, Rachel's mother went to a psychic who told her that both her children were spiritually gifted, even though she had never met Rachel or her brother. Rachel took both these incidents with a grain of salt, but they stayed with her.

RACHEL KNEW FROM childhood that she had Indigenous heritage through her paternal grandmother (her father's father was Ukrainian; her mother's heritage was Irish and Scottish). But she understood that due to the ongoing impacts of colonization, her grandmother had become disconnected from her birth culture and therefore never passed on the traditional knowledge and teachings that normally would be Rachel's father's—and Rachel's—birthright. Talking about the past was painful for her grandmother, so she didn't. And since the Chippewas of Georgina Island, the Anishinaabe Nation her grandmother was a member of, was headquartered a two-and-a-half-hour drive from KW on the shores of faraway Lake Simcoe, she couldn't just pop by. For the time being, there seemed no easy way back to her culture.

Rachel's identification as AnishinaabeKwe came through not in an *A-ha!* moment, but through a series of experiences. She was twenty when she got her status card. But status cards only prove that you're Indigenous in the eyes of the Canadian government. Truly being part of any Indigenous community, Rachel learned, requires more than a piece of plastic with a bad photo. Community is about reciprocity: the more you give to it, the more you get out of it.

It was at university that Rachel first got an inkling of what she'd been looking for all those years. While doing a communications degree at Carlton University in Ottawa, she got involved with the school's Indigenous Student Centre and took some courses in human rights and ancient history. Maybe answers to some of the big questions could be found in the past? Instead of answers, she learned how religion, including Catholicism, had been used by various societies as a tool for coercion. This didn't sit well with her. And it made her even more determined to figure out what did.

As a kid, she had wanted to be a vet, but she realized she loved animals too much to work with them in that way. She thought another "compassion profession" like nursing might suit her—her mother was a nurse—but when she spoke to her high school guidance counsellor about doing more math and sciences courses so she could get into a nursing program, he checked her grades and strongly discouraged her. He did not mention the many transition programs that exist to help people just like Rachel get the grades necessary to go into the professions that appeal to them.

Rachel found she didn't really enjoy communications (which had been the guidance counsellor's idea, not hers). She had three placements in government positions while she was in Ottawa, all of which she found dull and unproductive. Determined to get the high school credits she needed to pursue her true passion, and with her mom's encouragement, she enrolled in a general arts and sciences program at Conestoga College in KW. She did well. So well that she got early acceptance into an RPN program, which led to a Bachelor of Science in Nursing program at Ontario Tech in Oshawa, Ontario.

Like Carlton, both schools had Indigenous student centres. The difference was that Rachel now had both the time and the knowledge to take advantage of the supports and resources they offered. Through these centres, she accessed what felt like real community for the first time. Things snowballed from there. At Ontario Tech, the Indigenous Student Centre was run by a group of Indigenous women who took Rachel under their wing. They introduced her to community elders and encouraged her to get involved with Native youth. They guided and supported her and generally inspired her to get out of her comfort zone (something she says they continue to do to this day).

Like a lot of Indigenous people who have become disconnected from their culture, Rachel decided to make up for lost time by participating in traditional ceremonies, some of which were suppressed by the American and Canadian governments in the nineteenth and twentieth centuries. While doing an Indigenous research fellowship as part of her graduate studies, she met an elder who helped her embark on a berry fast, a rite of passage typically undertaken by a girl after her first period, known as the moon time. (Unlike many cultures that consider menstruation a curse, some First Nations groups look upon it as a time when girls become spiritually powerful.) The rite typically involves elder women teaching the girl undergoing it about self-control and the sacredness of the body. But it has also evolved over the years due to the effects of colonization to accommodate the needs of urban Indigenous people like Rachel. Since she wasn't an adolescent anymore, Rachel decided she would perform the rite for her inner child. Between October and the strawberry moon the following June, she abstained from eating all berries (a tall order, since Rachel loves them) or even anything berry flavoured. She took these strictures seriously. For instance, when she discovered that the ingredients in her multivitamin powder contained berries, she stopped using it.

As much as nursing school helped Rachel reconnect with her indigeneity, there were things there that bothered her. She found that when profs covered Indigenous topics they often leaned into stereotypes and provided little room for discussion about them. For example, the high incidence of diabetes among Indigenous people might get mentioned, but not the complicated reasons why, which include the fact that colonial institutions and practices like residential schools, Indian hospitals, and the Sixties Scoop all limited Indigenous people's access not just to their culture but also to nutritious and affordable food. (In addition, Indigenous people have a strong genetic risk for type 2 diabetes.) None of her classes covered traditional health, healing, or racism. They would approach cultural safe care once, tick a box, and never mention it again.

When these types of things didn't sit right with Rachel, or when she found herself coping with a power differential—it could be as basic as approaching a prof for a potential reference, or as complex as approaching someone who makes culturally inappropriate statements—she went to her group at the Indigenous centre, and the new sources they had put her in touch with, to talk about it. They invariably offered useful advice. But they also saw that Rachel had a natural gift for advocacy and encouraged her to keep using it.

She took this encouragement to heart. One of her earliest successes as an advocate was as a member of Nursing Students of Ontario, a student-governed interest group associated with the Registered Nurses' Association of Ontario (RNAO). She helped secure a permanent seat for Indigenous youth on the association's executive team. Later, she networked to get Indigenous elders and knowledge keepers to open a major conference she was helping to organize as a member of another student group with national reach, the Canadian Nursing Students' Association. The conference covered topics like the ongoing impact of colonization on healthcare; stereotyping; and the horrific practices— shockingly, still ongoing—of coerced and forced sterilization and birth alerts: where nurses notify hospitals and child welfare agencies to apprehend children right after they're born. Though Rachel was familiar with most of these things, hearing about them firsthand from Indigenous nurses was deeply impactful.

The conference brought home to Rachel just how much power nurses and other healthcare providers have in our society, even if they're not aware of it. Indigenous patients, on the other hand, especially those who've had bad personal experiences in hospitals or through intergenerational trauma, feel that power differential the second they walk through a hospital door.

Rachel's first job after graduating gave her a shot at changing this. As a patient navigator for Southwest Ontario Aboriginal Health Access Centre (SOAHAC), which runs Indigenous-led health clinics all over the province, her role would be to go into hospitals in the region and support any Indigenous patients who requested assistance (their families could request it too): moms with new babies, young adults with mental health issues, older folks getting surgery. Sometimes she'd get called in just to sit with an Indigenous person who'd gone into emerg. If the patient was admitted, she'd follow them ward to ward, if necessary. Doctors can be intimidating, so Rachel served as a kind of interpreter by simplifying confusing medical jargon for her clients. In addition to bridging cultural and linguistic gaps, she was also tasked with creating plans for ongoing patient care and discharge.

Because specialized hospital care tends to be located in dense urban areas, Indigenous patients often came long distances to access it. If their case was urgent, patients would often arrive alone on short notice without the supplies they'd normally pack, and with no family to support them. For these patients, Rachel would act as a kind of proxy for family, fetching whatever the patient wanted or needed to make them more comfortable, whether a toothbrush, a bottle of cranberry juice, or a magazine.

Helping her clients understand the system they were in was important, but Rachel often found that what they wanted the most was a fellow human being to interact with. This was especially crucial during Covid, when families couldn't access hospitals even if they were close by. Individuals all had different ways of responding to Rachel, but to perform her role to the best of her ability, she first needed to build a patient's trust. It wasn't enough to simply tell them she was Indigenous too. Trust could take time, although when patients found out about her other work in the community with SOAHAC, most warmed up pretty quickly. A number of patients expressed their deep appreciation of what Rachel's program had done for them. One woman hand-beaded some beautiful pins, which she mailed to Rachel after she got home. Others dropped off small anonymous gifts at a clinic that ended up at Rachel's station.

When the pandemic hit, Rachel was seconded from her navigator role to help with the vaccine rollout. Her responsibilities, which included educating community members and booking appointments for those unable to do so, felt daunting, and she was a bit nervous. But working in the clinic would turn out to be one of the best jobs she ever had. Things were well organized and she felt supported by other staff. The atmosphere wasn't super chaotic, like everything was on fire. Best of all, she found she could take the time to connect with clients, meet their families. Do the kind of nursing that nurses basically never get to do. Within the impersonal environment of a mass immunization clinic, she was able to create safe spaces for Indigenous clients by ensuring that they could perform traditional practices like smudging—one of whose many purposes is to get the person doing it into a positive frame of mind—or by offering bags of traditional medicines like sweetgrass, sage, cedar, and tobacco to anyone who came in. She coached non-Indigenous nurses on how to interact with Indigenous clients, telling them not to make assumptions about what they would or wouldn't want (not all Indigenous people smudge, for instance) or to question someone who self-identifies as Indigenous during screening.

Some of that advice came from personal experience. Rachel had been at the receiving end of such assumptions, albeit of a different kind. When the vaccine rollout first began, officials took a slow-release approach to make sure the system didn't get overwhelmed. The first shots went to the highest priority groups, people with low immunity, people on chemo, and elderly and First Nations people. The same process was used for boosters. But when Rachel went to a clinic to get a booster, the screener insisted she wasn't yet eligible. Rachel didn't want to have to spell things out; she knew she didn't look "Indigenous," but this nurse was leaving her no choice. "Did you not read my chart? I'm Indigenous," she told the nurse. "Oh," the screener replied nonchalantly, "I only read the top part."

Rachel got her booster, but the incident made her think about vulnerable community members who might not have the resources or educational background to advocate for themselves if they got the same kind of pushback. Many, she knew, would simply leave the clinic and never return. So when she wrote to the head of the clinic to explain what had happened, she took a constructive approach, saying she wanted to share the resources she had so the problem wouldn't reoccur with future clients.

At their own vaccine clinic, the feedback Rachel got from Indigenous clients was overwhelmingly positive. Many said that having an

Indigenous person immunizing them had been really important. And they also liked that the process hadn't been cold and impersonal. Those who wanted to could get their shot in the usual three minutes, or have a half-hour chat with Rachel about where they were from or how they were feeling that day. They could also go through the regular line (not all Indigenous people were sent to her; it was their choice). "It's those relationship-building interactions that are going to make healthcare feel like a safer space for Indigenous folks going forward," Rachel says.

Though she acknowledges there's still a steep hill to climb to make healthcare truly accessible to all First Nations, Rachel believes things are at least going in the right direction. In the early days of Covid, when she was still a navigator and her unit was on lockdown, she got special permission from a hospital to temporarily disable the smoke alarm in the room of her client, an Indigenous woman who was there for cardiac surgery and wanted to smudge beforehand (smudging was allowed at the hospital, but it was usually done in a different space). Accommodations like this—and the fact that the hospital even had smudge kits available for patients—would have been almost unthinkable just a decade ago.

Healthcare providers' attitudes to Indigenous patients are often the result of a lack of education and training rather than outright racism. Rachel started to realize this when hospital staff asked her with genuine curiosity why her navigator role was necessary. Didn't all Indigenous people live on reserves? Over time, Rachel's constant presence on the wards showed them that this wasn't the case (in Canada, 75 percent of Indigenous people live off-reserve, but they face just as much racism).

RACHEL SPENDS SOME of her time these days speaking to future nurses about Indigenous health at schools and workshops. In March 2023, she was the only nurse on a five-woman delegation sent by Young Diplomats of Canada to deliver an oral statement at the sixty-seventh Commission on the Status of Women at the United Nations in New York.

Most nursing programs, if they haven't done so already, are in the process of developing Indigenous health courses in response to 2015's landmark Truth and Reconciliation Commission, which called on medical and nursing schools in Canada "to require all students to take a course dealing with Aboriginal health issues, including the history and legacy of residential schools, the United Nations Declaration on the Rights of Indigenous Peoples, Treaties and Aboriginal rights, and Indigenous teachings and practices." Rachel finds it a bit problematic that the courses are still being delivered through colonial institutions. She would like to see more consultation and input from Indigenous communities and staff during course creation. But she sees it as a hopeful start to a longer process. "If truth and reconciliation could be achieved in healthcare with just a simple course, it would have been done by now."

A Call to Arms

*B*ack in 2019, *we* were both in a dark place. Our nursing "dream jobs" were making us feel silenced, gaslighted, and defeated, and our mental health was in a precarious state.

In order to cope, we talked to each other every day on speakerphone during our 35-minute commutes home. It helped us decompress and feel less alone.

We knew we weren't the only ones who felt this way. We were sure that other nurses would benefit from the kinds of cathartic conversations the two of us were lucky enough to share. But how could we expand the experience beyond our cars? We dreamed of creating a community of nurses who would empower one another and—who knows?—maybe even find solutions to our continued marginalization in the healthcare sphere.

At the time, Amie's cousin Sandy Hudson, a co-founder of Black Lives Matter Canada, and her close friend Nora Loreto were hosting a successful weekly podcast called *Sandy and Nora Talk Politics*. When

Amie asked Sandy what she enjoyed about the podcast, she answered unequivocally: the opportunity to freely express her opinions and shine light on political issues that might otherwise get ignored.

Could two nurses with no public profile do something similar?

Who was going to stop us if we tried?

WE KNEW WE wanted to create a podcast where we shared our thoughts—the good, the bad, and the ugly—about our chosen field. But what to call it? A word that kept popping up after our ordeal with the abusive administrator (described in the chapters "The Making of a Gritty Nurse: Sara" and "The Making of a Gritty Nurse: Amie"), was *resiliency*. She'd made us feel that we *weren't* resilient. But we knew that wasn't true. In fact, we knew we had more than resilience—we had *grit*. The word resonated, and so *The Gritty Nurse Podcast* was born.

It was a grey Sunday in December 2019 when we cracked open laptops in our respective homes and launched the free Audacity software we had downloaded. We had no notes, just our shaky voices and off-the-cuff opinions. Technically, we were winging it (at the end of our first episode you'll hear one of us saying, "How do we turn this off?"). It was no coincidence that our episodes were about the same length as our car speaker phone conversations. They still are.

Nervousness aside, there was no pressure. Although we still had our respective post-abusive administrator jobs, the podcast itself wasn't affiliated with any institution or organization. And it's not like anyone was listening. After we posted our first episode, we were thrilled to see we'd gotten thirty downloads. That meant thirty people wanted to hear what we had to say!

The possibility that *The Gritty Nurse Podcast* might one day top the podcast charts and gain an international audience, or that we'd eventually be sharing our thoughts on healthcare issues with a national broadcast audience across six time zones couldn't have been further from our minds or expectations. Had we known where the path we had tentatively set foot on would lead us, we might never have taken it in the first place.

A FEW MONTHS after our launch the pandemic hit, and so by necessity our focus changed. You could say we were in the right place at the right time, even if that time was a painful one. Hospitals were critically short-staffed because nurses were burning out, quitting, even dying. Nursing students were being fast-tracked to graduate, but not fast enough.

The murder of George Floyd in the summer of 2020 was another pivot point. The conversation about racism was becoming global. What about racism in nursing? What about women's rights and women's health? What about issues within the profession that nurses rarely talk about, like lateral nursing violence and sexual harassment, not to mention socio-political issues, mental health, and nursing's public image?

As the crisis deepened, we consumed media coverage and asked, Where are the nurses in all this? The province of Ontario had set up a Covid-19 task force that included the recently retired Toronto chief of police but, mind-bogglingly, no nurses. (The federal task force at least had *one* nurse.) It was obvious that the public and the media didn't understand what the role of nurses was in the crisis, or what it could be. This was nothing new. When it comes to decision-making in health-care, nurses have rarely had a voice or agency, but all the talk about nurses being the heroes of the pandemic, all the banging of pots and pans, made the system's indifference to us extra hard to take.

On January 5, 2021, a CBC producer reached out. Could we do a live interview with Andrew Nichols on national TV about nurses' potential role in the (then) floundering provincial vaccine rollout? At that point, we had just over a year of podcasting under our belts, but we were basically working in a vacuum. We had no media training (who, exactly, would train us?). And we'd both heard boogeyman stories of nurses who had been punished for appearing in the media. Would that be us? Maybe. But we made the decision any gritty nurse would make: to do it anyway.

The caption that ran over the seven-minute interview read **We're Ready to Help,** which was indeed our message. Overall, the interview went well, although afterwards we both agreed that—aside from childbirth and workplace bullying—it was the scariest experience either of us had ever had.

Our appearance on Andrew Nichols's show was the exception, not the rule. Nurses were not considered to be experts or people who had anything to contribute. Though we were big fans of Dr. Brian Goldman's CBC Radio show, *White Coat, Black Art,* for instance, it was impossible not to notice that nurses were not included in the show's discussions on the pandemic. After a while, listening to physicians continually speak on our behalf became too much. Pointing out that we didn't have a seat at the Covid decision-making table, we tweeted at Dr. Goldman: "We are ready and willing! Lives are at stake. There are so many willing to help. You just have to ask."

Dr. Goldman, to his credit, reached out almost immediately, and just over a week later we did a segment on *White Coat, Black Art* that touched on systemic racism in healthcare and vaccine hesitancy during the rollout.

Our appearance on the show seemed to open the floodgates. Requests for interviews poured in and basically never stopped, even as the pandemic waned. Suddenly, our small but loyal audience, which consisted mainly of other nurses and healthcare professionals, was expanding into the general public.

We've tried to use each of those appearances (there have been hundreds, on every major Canadian network), as well as opinion pieces for magazines and newspapers, to bring attention to the short- and long-term issues affecting nurses and healthcare. (One advantage of being a duo is that whenever there's a media request, one of us is generally available to do it. We divide and conquer!)

We've never claimed we have answers to all the problems facing nursing or healthcare. Our goal has always been to start conversations. Based on the feedback we get from listeners, public figures, and people we reconnected with from our early days of nursing, it feels like we've accomplished that. Nursing professors tell us that they recommend our podcast to their students. Some of them even use episodes in their assignments. People we don't know recognize us in the street and tell us how much they love the podcast. It's surreal, but also gratifying.

NURSING HAS ALWAYS been essential work, even if it took a global pandemic for people to recognize it. We are among the few professionals that are present at the beginning and the end of life—not to mention at all the times in between—and on the best and worst days. Are nurses the backbone of the healthcare system? We think we're more like the heart of it.

Starting an IV, dressing a wound, or giving an injection: nurses are so much more than the lists of tasks we perform. We're the hand the patient holds when they're in pain, the encouraging voice that gets a woman through childbirth, the shoulder to cry on when you receive a devastating diagnosis or a loved one passes away.

We're the ones that spend the most time with patients when everyone else in the hospital seems to be coming and going. And because we spend so much time with them, we're often their best advocates. Our cumulative experience is the source of our wisdom (that, plus years of intense study).

For that same reason, we're also the best advocates for ourselves and our profession. As a group, we have agency. Our "gentle hands" can braid your hair in the ICU, but when it comes to protecting our healthcare system, they can also hoist a placard as we march in the streets.

And yet our voices and wisdom have too often been excluded from the healthcare conversation. The mainstream view of nursing, baked in from Florence Nightingale days, often continues to be one of subservience, as simply a "helper" to physicians.

It's time to finally break the stereotypes. We aren't sexy nurses. We aren't Nurse Ratched. We're not meek handmaidens to doctors. Nursing is more diverse than ever before, both the people doing it and the kinds of jobs available—there are literally hundreds, way more than can be listed in this book (go on, google it). Nurses today are changemakers, leaders, and advocates. They're even shaking things up in non-traditional areas such as politics, as hospital CEOs, as consultants, as heads of major organizations. Nursing education is changing for the better too, albeit slowly.

WE NURSES ARE still due for a reckoning within the profession. Tone policing, respectability politics, morality-based hiring—all these need to stop. If we don't have respect and solidarity within our own profession, how can we ask others to respect us and stand with us?

So how do we bring about change?

If you're a nurse, then get a seat at the table. We can't tell you how many times we've called individuals and healthcare organizations out for not seeking nurse input on issues that affect nurses. It seems like common sense, but you'd be surprised how often it happens. If the issue concerns nursing, ask yourself if you've heard a nurse's perspective. If you haven't, consider being the one to offer that perspective.

Of course, having a seat at the table is not the same as having actual power to make change. We've been at tables where it was clear that we functioned as tokens, and all the important decisions had been made in advance. We need more nurses in permanent nursing chief officer roles, in politics, in home and community healthcare. Again, ask yourself: Could that be me?

But you don't have to be a nurse, a healthcare professional, or an influencer to enact change. Anyone can help make healthcare better by showing up at a rally or a protest, posting on social media, writing an email to their local politician, or just saying thank you to a nurse (we remember it).

When you stand up for nurses, you're standing up for better health outcomes for yourself and your family. We do this work because we care deeply for people, so if you care for us back, well . . . think of it as good karma.

SANDY HUDSON WAS right: the most fulfilling thing about what we do is having the freedom to say what we really think. Neither of us feels constrained or intimidated by anyone anymore.

We've learned that, at our core, the two of us are advocates and storytellers. That's why we started *The Gritty Nurse Podcast* and why we wrote this book. Nursing's image has been stuck in amber for over a century. We'd like to think we're helping the image to break out.

Neither of us knows where this journey will lead. What we do know is that the conversation around nursing needs to continue. In many ways it's just beginning.

So let's start again.

Can you name a famous nurse?

ACKNOWLEDGEMENTS

This book would not be possible without the help of so many people who kindly shared their stories, encouraged us, and helped us along the way. Our immense thanks to Rick Broadhead, Emily Donaldson, Brad Wilson and the team at HarperCollins, Dr. Brian Goldman, Dr. Leigh Chapman, Dr. Alika La Fontaine, CBC News, Tim Guest, Dr. Michelle Acorn, Swardiq Mayanja, Nikki Skillen, Cathy Crowe, Dr. Natalie Stake-Doucet, David Metzger, Lindsay Pentland, Matthew Shepherd, Rachel Radyk, Adrienne Behning, the National Speakers Bureau, Reshmi Nair, and the U of T Lawrence Bloomberg School of Nursing.

Thanks too to all the patients who impacted our lives and shared their journey with us, all the listeners of *The Gritty Nurse Podcast*, and every single one of you nurses out there for sharing your grit and nursing wisdom.